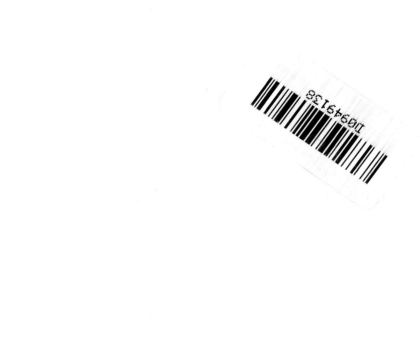

Naturally Healthy Kids

Integrating Conventional and Holistic Treatments for Common Illnesses of Children

Jerry Rubin MD   **Dean Prina** MD
Nancy Lataitis MD   **Jordan R. Klein** MD

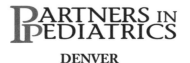

DENVER

www.naturallyhealthykids.com

Publisher's Cataloging-in-Publication

Naturally healthy kids : integrating conventional and
    holistic treatments for common illnesses of children /
    Jerry Rubin ... [et al.].
    p. cm.
    LCCN 2006900795
    ISBN-13: 9780977394920
    ISBN-10: 0977394921

    1. Pediatrics--Popular works. 2. Infants--Health and
hygiene--Popular works. 3. Children--Health and hygiene
--Popular works. 4. Children--Diseases--Alternative
treatment--Popular works.   I. Rubin, Jerry, 1951-

RJ61.N343 2006   618.92
                         QBI06-600046

Production Management by
Paros Press
1551 Larimer Street, Suite 1301   Denver, CO 80202
303-893-3332   www.parospress.com

Book Design by Scott Johnson

Printed in the United States of America
1 3 5 7 9 10 8 6 4 2

TABLE OF CONTENTS

INTRODUCTION

What makes this book different from others available today?

We combine advice from our traditional, western medicine training as M.D.'s with information from practicing a more holistic approach to children's health. We believe we are among a very small group of physicians nationally who are on the cutting edge of safely combining many health modalities.

A real desire exists among parents to treat their children more naturally and to avoid any side effects from medicine. By embracing a fuller spectrum of health care options, we have discovered that not only can some natural treatments be curative, but also preventive. And we have learned much from our patients, who have shared their personal experiences with healthy natural solutions.

This book is our fourth and by far most comprehensive revision of a guide we have been publishing for our patients for years. We never dreamed we'd publish a book for national distribution. But then again, when we started our practice nearly thirty years ago, we never would have predicted today's unprecedented interest in and demand for a more natural approach to serving children.

Our natural treatments have given us additional tools for our "doctor's bag." Trust us and our experience caring for children. And trust yourself to make natural choices for your children's health.

Our patients consider this book a most valuable resource. We appreciate their approval, confidence, and suggestions. You'll find this book easy to read, easy to reference, and clearly organized.

In Health,

Jerry Rubin, M.D.
Dean Prina, M.D.
Nancy Lataitis, M.D.
Jordan R. Klein, M.D.

We gratefully acknowledge the support and wisdom of all the providers and staff of Partners in Pediatrics.

We have designed this handbook to be your **most accurate** and useful home illness guide. Please take a few minutes now to familiarize yourself with its general format for your easy reference. The first section contains a table of contents alphabetized according to symptoms or illnesses. It also contains general information about integrated medicine, and general principles of medical support.

The second section contains four guides for quick and easy reference.

☞ The first one gives exact guidance on the doses of commonly used over-the-counter medications.

☞ The second one contains all information regarding methods of administering and dosing aromatherapy, herbal, homeopathic, and nutritional therapies.

☞ The third one is a complete list of herbal and homeopathic products. Guidance for the use of these products is referenced in the "Integrated Therapies" portion of each illness section.

☞ The fourth one covers the most important aspects of common first aid.

In the third section there are a number of illnesses or symptoms described in detail to guide you in home health care. This information will give you the guidance to initiate health-care measures to support and nurture your child through that illness. Illnesses **always** have a spectrum of intensity. The guidance in the handbook is designed for children experiencing **mild to moderate** forms of the disorder.

You will notice that each symptom/illness section begins with a description of the problem or symptom (with pertinent information about physiology, causes, expected course, and contagiousness), followed by home management guidelines and our integrated health-care advice, directions about when to call your health-care provider, references to other similar topics, and tips on prevention.

We have carefully included all of the common recommendations, from both conventional and integrated health-care disciplines, that we have seen benefit children over our many years of experience. In many cases there **may be more than one suggestion** to accomplish the same goal (for example, several different creams for itching). When more than one option appears in the same section, you may use whichever one **best fits** your needs at the time. In deciding, you might take into account your own previous experiences (level of benefit, side effects), product availability (try to use things you have on hand), your child's anticipated compliance (taste, ease, and frequency of administration), and your own intuition. You may also very comfortably **mix** conventional and integrated options (unless otherwise noted) to optimally support your child through an illness, but it is also important to keep your program as simple as possible. If you try an option and it doesn't work or your child refuses to take it, you may want to review the section again and select another option. There is no single best recipe to manage any illness that applies to **all** children, and no substitute for your own personal experience regarding what your child will or will not respond to. You are strongly encouraged to explore new options. **Through careful observation, your experience and intuition will serve you powerfully in refining your approach to find the most effective treatment for your child.**

To enhance your ability to treat your child at home, we recommend that you keep a basic supply of all the common medications, herbals, homeopathics, etc., that you use or may need to have on hand.

INTEGRATED MEDICINE

Health care is changing rapidly and so are the terms we use to describe health-care practices. When our office first opened in 1977 the term "integrated" medicine did not exist, nor did "holistic," "complementary," or "alternative" medicine. Many health-care practices, such as acupuncture, have enjoyed great success and popularity for centuries in cultures other than our own. Many of these practices have stood up well to the scientific scrutiny of conventional medicine.

"Integrated medicine" is the term we have selected to best describe how we practice modern medicine. "Integrated medicine" might be defined as **preventive-oriented medicine that considers the whole person** (body, mind, spirit, social, and lifestyle) in evaluating health-care needs. It emphasizes a partnership and makes use of all appropriate therapies—conventional, complementary, and alternative—to maintain or regain one's health. We chose this phrase because it captures how we use conventional medical therapies and integrate them with other forms of health-care practices such as homeopathy, nutritional supplementation, etc.

Medical doctors have traditionally viewed these other treatments as if they were in opposition to conventional medicine. Doctors are only now breaking through the barriers of that perspective to genuinely evaluate the potential benefits of these non-conventional methods as valid "alternatives" for healing that "complement" conventional care. More and more **doctors are learning how to successfully incorporate both approaches** into the everyday practice of medicine. It is beyond the scope of this handbook to comprehensively list all forms of non-conventional care, but for the convenience of this discussion, we have organized them into several categories and have limited the examples to some of the best-known therapies.

1. BODY WORK
   A. CHIROPRACTIC
   B. OSTEOPATHIC
   C. MASSAGE THERAPY
   D. YOGA

2. BIOENERGETIC
   A. ACUPUNCTURE
   B. REIKI
   C. BIO-FEEDBACK
   D. HOMEOPATHIC MEDICINE **
   E. BACH FLOWER THERAPY **

3. BIOMOLECULAR
   A. CONVENTIONAL MEDICINE **
   B. HERBAL THERAPIES**
   C. NUTRITIONAL SUPPLEMENTS **
   D. DIETARY THERAPY **
   E. AROMATHERAPY**

** These are therapies we use in our integrated approach.

OVERVIEW OF INTEGRATED MODALITIES

The following is a brief overview for your education and interest. We hope it will enhance your utilization of the handbook.

CONVENTIONAL MEDICINE

Conventional medicine is known by a variety of names, including **Western medicine, Allopathic medicine, and Orthodox medicine.** Conventional medicine is the most common form of health care practiced in the United States, and has been for nearly a century. The popularity and acceptance of western medicine was built upon **three very powerful tools**:

1. Astonishing advances in **surgery, anesthesia, and pain management** have transformed surgery from a "last resort" method in life-threatening events to a viable, effective, and often minimally invasive technique. Cesarean sections, for example, have dramatically improved the safety of childbearing.

2. **Diagnostic methodologies, including blood chemistry and radiographic imaging, are one of conventional medicine's most powerful groups of tools.** The ability to rapidly and accurately assess harmful changes in blood chemistry balance has allowed early and successful interventions in heart, lung, and fluid abnormalities as well as early diagnosis of serious diseases such as cancer. New advances in radiographic imaging allow rapid, accurate, and detailed assessments in a non-invasive way with minimal to no exposure to radiation. This arena alone has revolutionized both the safety and efficacy of conventional medicine.

3. Perhaps the greatest set of tools, however, that propelled conventional medicine to the forefront of health care in this country was the advent of the **ability to control and treat infectious diseases with antibiotics and the ability to prevent some with vaccines.** It is difficult for us to com-

prehend the impact of this single aspect of conventional medicine when just 70 years ago widespread panic surrounded the tragic loss from an epidemic of scarlet fever or polio, now considered diseases of the past.

Conventional medicine has its roots in ancient Greek medicine and Hippocrates, who taught that the diagnosis could often be made by listening carefully to the patient's story. He believed that close evaluation of the patient's diet, habits, emotions, occupation, stresses and climate tolerance, along with close observation for changes in physical appearance (for example, swelling), coupled with logical reasoning, would allow the physician to determine the cause of an illness and so point to its cure. This approach formed the foundation for our modern-day history and physical examination.

Today, conventional medicine faces some challenges. The scientific approach of conventional medicine encourages protocols and objectification of therapy, which can diminish the intuitive and creative participation of parents and health-care providers in nurturing the patient back to health. Physicians and parents must also be careful not to diminish their careful observations by over-reliance on the powerful investigative tools of conventional medicine. The **overuse of antibiotics is creating resistant strains of bacteria.** The powerful effects of many drugs can be overshadowed by their side effects and the fact that they often suppress symptoms without curing diseases.

We believe that conventional medicine can be more powerful than ever if its great strengths and advances in technology are balanced by careful listening and observation and further enhanced by the use of the many safe, gentle, and effective methods of complementary health-care systems as discussed below.

AROMATHERAPY

Contrary to popular belief that aromatherapy uses fragrance to make things smell nice, aromatherapy is actually an **ancient art that uses the healing power of essential oils.** Essential oils are derived through distillation from a variety of plants. Of course, essential oils are used commercially for fragrances (for example, perfumes and candles) and flavorings (for example, vanilla extract). When they are used for these purposes the qualities of taste and aroma are more important than purity. For that reason they are often adjusted to suit the needs of the product.

However, essential oils have also been valued for thousands of years for their healing and medicinal properties. Here it is very important that they are produced and maintained with purity. There are many brands of essential oils on the market, and we recommend that you use only those considered **"therapeu-**

tic grade." This information should be available where you purchase the essential oils.

Essential oils, when administered correctly, are considered to have a wide variety of therapeutic benefits, including antiseptic, insect-repellant, calming, and sedating. The **advantages of aromatherapy are that essential oils are therapeutically effective and very safe, inexpensive, and well accepted by children.** There are two main ways essential oils can be administered in children: through inhalation and by topical (skin) application.

HERBAL REMEDIES

Herbal remedies use the healing properties of a variety of plants to help patients regain and maintain their health and well-being. Herbs have been used as a health resource for thousands of years. Although herbal remedies are often viewed by modern medicine as experimental and non-scientific, they are scientifically grounded and closely intertwined with conventional medicine. In fact, **it is estimated that over half of all drugs in modern conventional medicine today have their origins as an herbal remedy.** For example, the herb foxglove is the source of the modern drug digitalis, a medicine for heart failure. Herbalists used white willow bark for fever and pain relief long before pharmacologists developed its extract, aspirin. In fact, the line is so thin between conventional and herbal treatments that most of us would think of using prunes for constipation before taking a laxative.

Conventional pharmacological research seeks to isolate and study a single, active ingredient of a plant for its potential therapeutic benefits. **The herbalist believes that the healing properties of plants come from more than just their active ingredients.** The entire plant contains a wide variety of biochemical ingredients that enhance and support the active herbal ingredient, as well as safeguard against toxicity. When modern methods were developed by pharmaceutical laboratories to extract, purify, or synthesize active ingredients of healing plants, the use of herbs began to wane. The public began to favor the more "scientific" approach of drugs.

The science of herbology is substantially more complex than simply deciding which herb to use for which disorder. For example, herbalists have very specific criteria concerning when to harvest each plant to optimize its potency and which parts of the plant (for example, stem, leaf, root, or fruit) are to be used in the preparation of an herbal remedy. In addition, herbalists must also be able to determine the most effective herbal remedy, the exact dose, and the frequency of doses for each unique illness.

There are **several advantages to using herbal treatment.** For example, many herbal remedies support bodily functions for which there is not yet a conventional drug equivalent. In addition, because herbs contain a variety of supportive ingredients and often less of the potent active ingredient, they can be gentler than their drug equivalents. On the other hand, the therapeutic benefit of herbs is often slower than drugs, giving an advantage to drugs. **Herbs and drugs share one common theme, however: they are both active, biomolecular products, with effects and side effects.** Both must be used as intended, with wisdom and appropriate supervision.

Herbs are available as single remedies or in compounds that use several herbs to accomplish a more complex therapeutic goal. They are available in a variety of preparations, the most common of which include teas, tinctures, glycerites, syrups, capsules, tablets, and topical agents (salves, creams, gels, etc.).

Liquid extracts are concentrated extracts of the herb, obtained by soaking the herb in a liquid extractant. From a therapeutic point of view, they are the most potent way to administer an herbal remedy. A **tincture** is a liquid extract in which alcohol is used as the extractant. Tinctures have a very strong and frequently bad taste. They may also contain significant amounts of alcohol. These traits make them less favorable for use in infants and young children. A **glycerite** is a liquid extract in which glycerine, a sweet-tasting material derived from vegetable oil, is used as the extractant. Because glycerites are far better tasting and free of alcohol, they are a much better therapeutic choice for children.

Capsules and tablets are also popular and convenient ways of administering herbs. The primary advantage of capsules is their convenience of administration. The major disadvantage of capsules is that they are less potent than tinctures. Also, a young child may not be able to swallow a capsule.

Herbal teas are readily available and come in a wide variety. Herbal teas in tea bags are considered beverage teas because the concentration of herb in the tea is typically too diluted to be therapeutic. There is no doubt, however, that a cup of chamomile tea can soothe and comfort an ill or stressed child. A properly prepared infusion of the loose herbs, however, is considered a very effective and easy way to administer herbal remedies to children.

Topical agents such as creams, salves, and gels have also entered into mainstream use; for example, we are all familiar with using aloe vera for burns.

On some occasions, for example before surgery, we may recommend avoidance of particular oral herbal therapies. Be sure to discuss their use with your health-care provider.

HOMEOPATHY

Homeopathy is a scientific approach to health care that was founded more than 200 years ago by German physician Dr. Samuel Hahnemann. Hahnemann rediscovered a medical principle first put forth by Hippocrates known as **"the law of similars," which roughly states that a substance (remedy) that creates a certain set of symptoms in a healthy person would be able to cure a person who has an illness with the same set of symptoms.**

Hahnemann began his studies by first testing his hypothesis on himself and his close friends. These tests were called **"provings"** and involved taking small amounts of a certain substance and observing and recording every change in his patients' physical, mental, and emotional make-up, regardless of how slight the change might be. He then discovered that when he diluted the same substance to an infinitesimal amount, it would cure the same symptom pattern that he had observed in the "proving." His results were remarkably successful and reproducible. **Hahnemann demonstrated that a homeopathic remedy can cure a disease in which the symptoms are similar to the reaction it would create if the remedy were to be administered to a healthy person.** In other words, **"the like cures the like."** This is where the word homeopathy derives its meaning, from the Greek homios, which means "similar," and pathy, which means "suffering."

Homeopathy differs in many ways from conventional medicine, but one of its primary differences is that homeopathy seeks to find the **unique "imprint" of the disease symptom** as it manifests in an individual. Rather than diagnosing the disease by seeking the cause (for example, an infectious agent) as in conventional medicine, homeopathy seeks to diagnose the disease through the unique pattern of symptoms; then the homeopathic remedy is selected and administered to stimulate a resolution of the illness.

Since Hahnemann's time, **over 3,000 homeopathic remedies have been tested through "provings."** The majority of these remedies are derived from plant materials (approximately 80 percent), with most of the remaining substances coming from minerals (approximately 20 percent), and only a very small amount from animals.

Homeopathic remedies are prepared by a process called potentization. This process involves a series of **dilutions of the original "mother tincture" of the substance.** A mother tincture is an alcohol-based extract of the remedy (the original substance) and is similar to an herbal tincture. When the mother tincture is diluted one part in ten, it is called an "x" potency, and when it is diluted one part in a hundred, it is called a "c" potency. There will be a number in front of the "x" or "c," which indicates the number of times the tincture has been taken through such a dilution. Thus, a 5x potency means that the original tincture has been diluted one part in ten and then this new dilution is further diluted one part in ten, and the process is repeated a total of 5 times.

The fewer times that a remedy is diluted, the less potent it is; therefore, a homeopathic remedy at 5x is less potent than 10x even though the 5x is a "stronger" concentration. Thus, the fewer the molecules of mother tincture remaining in the diluted remedy, the more powerful the effect. The mechanism by which this occurs is unknown, but it would indicate that **homeopathic remedies do not work through traditional biomolecular models as do conventional drugs and herbal medicines.** This mystery is a possible explanation of why homeopathy is so gentle and safe. It is also one reason that many conventional physicians dismiss homeopathy as a legitimate therapy.

Originally, homeopathic remedies were administered by giving one remedy in one potency, one time, and then waiting weeks to determine the results. This is known as **"classic" homeopathy.** Classic homeopathy is best suited for serious or chronic diseases, but it requires a lengthy history to determine the correct remedy that fits the patient's exact profile of symptoms.

Over the past 50 years, modern research in homeopathy has led to new methods of using homeopathic remedies. **"Modern" homeopathy** now uses several different remedies and/or several potencies (all low potencies) of the same remedy in the same dose and uses doses several times per day. One of the primary advantages of this method is that it allows a remedy to be designed for a specific conventional diagnosis or symptom—for example, cough. This is the primary method of homeopathy that we use in our practice.

BACH FLOWER REMEDIES

English physician, bacteriologist, and homeopath, Edward Bach, developed the Bach Flower system. Dr. Bach believed that changes in emotional health could lead to physical disorders. He discovered that **preparations derived from flowering plants could restore a patient's emotional balance** and, in the process, frequently resolve physical symptoms. For example, we have all had the experience of an emotional upset triggering nausea or diarrhea, which then resolves when emotional balance returns.

There are **38 individual remedies in the Bach Flower system.** Each remedy addresses a specific emotional **"imbalance" such as fear, anxiety, self-absorption, strong will, etc.** There is also a 39th Bach Flower remedy known as Rescue Remedy™, which is a blend of 5 of the original 38 remedies and is specifically designed for stress management.

Dr. Bach's **flower essences are similar to homeopathic remedies** in that the mother tincture is often diluted prior to administration, but the **flower essences** may also be given in their undiluted form.

A Bach Flower treatment usually consists of selecting several individual remedies that address a larger profile of the patient's emotional health and placing them all in a single mixture. In addition, they can be useful in acute illnesses to quiet intense emotions. This is primarily how we use Bach Flower remedies in this handbook. They are also extremely useful in more chronic conditions not discussed in this handbook (for example, insomnia, behavioral management, phobias, etc.).

DIET AND NUTRITIONAL SUPPLEMENTATION

The history of making dietary changes to help heal a patient is as old as medicine itself. We are all familiar with avoiding coffee for patients with ulcers and increasing fiber for those with constipation.

More recent advances have allowed us to isolate or synthesize a wide array of specific nutrients—for example, vitamin C. These nutrients can be used alone or be combined with other nutrients such as calcium and magnesium, as dietary supplements. **Nutrient supplements can be used to simply ensure that the body has a basic supply of nutrients to optimize normal functions** (such as a daily multivitamin and multi-mineral supplement). **Nutrient supplements may also be used to enhance or intensify a specific function of the body;** for example, zinc and/or vitamin C may help to ward off a common cold.

Scientific controversy exists about whether or not a specific nutrient has any measurable benefit (for example, does vitamin C really affect colds?). We believe that, regardless of unresolved controversies, nutrient supplements and dietary changes, when used safely, may support and enhance the body's ability to protect and repair itself from a variety of stresses. This belief forms the basis for the recommendations in our handbook.

OVER-THE-COUNTER (OTC) MEDICATION RECOMMENDATIONS AND DOSAGES

Our philosophy for the use of over-the-counter medications is that they be used only when relief of symptoms is necessary to promote adequate comfort and rest for your child.

GENERAL SUGGESTIONS:

1. **Do not use other children's prescription medications or ANY ADULT medication** without first consulting your health-care provider.

2. **Do not use "leftover antibiotics" at any time. Improper use of antibiotics may:**
   - interfere with your health-care provider's ability to obtain an accurate diagnosis or test (for example, a rapid strep test/culture may be falsely negative if your child has been "pretreated" with antibiotics).
   - lead to reactions such as hives, vomiting, and diarrhea, which may complicate diagnosis and treatment as well as your child's recovery.
   - contribute to the increasing problem of "antibiotic resistance," making it more difficult to treat your child's subsequent bacterial infections.

3. Always **check expiration dates** before using medications.

4. Remember that infants and children are not "little adults" when it comes to medication dosing. Many ingredients in adult medications can be harmful to children.

5. Generic forms of medication may be substituted (such as ibuprofen for Motrin® or Advil®).

6. You may try natural preparations first for more gentle relief of symptoms (see individual sections for suggestions) before using over-the-counter medications.

7. **Use an ACCURATE measuring spoon, dropper, or syringe** when dosing your child. (TIP: 1 teaspoon = 5cc or 5ml)

8. **NEVER USE ANY ASPIRIN-CONTAINING MEDICATION** in children.

FOR DISCOMFORT AND IRRITABILITY ASSOCIATED WITH FEVER

ACETAMINOPHEN DOSING (Tylenol ®, Feverall ®)
May administer every 4 hours

WEIGHT	Infant drops (80mg/0.8ml)	Suspension (160 mg/5ml)	Chewable tab (80 mg)	Capsule/Tab (325 mg)	Rectal Suppository*
up to 6 lbs	0.4 ml	1/4 tsp	-	-	-
6 - 9 lbs	0.6 ml	3/8 tsp	-	-	-
9 - 12 lbs	0.8 ml	1/2 tsp	-	-	one 80 mg
12 - 18 lbs	1.2 ml	3/4 tsp	-	-	one 120 mg
18 - 24 lbs	1.6 ml	1 tsp	2	-	120 mg
24 - 35 lbs	2.4 ml	1 1/2 tsp	3	-	1/2 of 320 mg
35 - 47 lbs	-	2 tsp	4	1	one 320 mg
47 - 70 lbs	-	2 1/2 tsp	5	1	320 mg
70 - 95 lbs	-	3 tsp	6	1 1/2 (or one 500 mg "extra strength")	1 1/2 320 mg
> 95 lbs	-	-	-	2	two 320 mg

*A rectal suppository form of acetaminophen is also available without a prescription. This method of dosing may be preferable if vomiting, stomach irritation, or taste refusal occurs. Different strengths are available. Check above chart or package insert for dosing instructions.

These recommended doses are FOR PRODUCTS WHICH CONTAIN ONLY ACETAMINOPHEN. **Do not use the above chart for dosing combination products such as Tylenol Sinus®, etc.** Acetaminophen may be given along with antibiotics, decongestants, antihistamines, natural products and any other "multi-system relief" product that does NOT already contain acetaminophen. (**NOTE: In general, we do not recommend the use of multi-drug formulations** as their use may lead to under- or over-dosage for your child's symptoms).

IBUPROFEN DOSING (Motrin®, Advil®)
May be administered every 6 - 8 hours
The use of **ibuprofen IS NOT RECOMMENDED for**
infants less than 6 months of age.

WEIGHT	Infant drops (50mg/1.25ml)	Liquid (100mg/5ml)	Chewable tabs (50mg)	Tablets (100mg)	Tablet/Capsule (200mg)
12 - 18 lbs	1.25 ml	$1/2$ tsp	-	-	-
18 - 24 lbs	2.5 ml	1 tsp	1 - 2	-	-
24 - 35 lbs	3.75 ml	1 - $1^1/2$ tsp	2 - 3	1	-
35 - 47 lbs	-	2 tsp	3 - 4	$1^1/2$ - 2	-
47 - 66 lbs	-	2 - $2^1/2$ tsp	4 - 5	2 - 3	1
66 - 88 lbs	-	3 - $3^1/2$ tsp	6 - 7	3	1 - 2
> 88 lbs	-	4 tsp	8	4	2

These recommended doses are for products that contain only IBUPROFEN. **Do NOT use this dosing chart for combination medications (for example, Advil Cold®, etc.).** Ibuprofen may be given along with antibiotics, decongestants, antihistamines, natural products, or any other product that does NOT already contain ibuprofen (see above "NOTE"). To help alleviate stomach irritation, **give ibuprofen with food if possible.** In children over 100 lbs. and 10 yrs. or older, Aleve®, a non-steroidal anti-inflammatory with longer duration of action, may be used in place of ibuprofen TWICE a day or every 12 hours for pain relief (for dosing guidelines follow the package inserts).
NOTE: For treatment of persistent discomfort, you may alternate the dosing of ibuprofen with a dose of acetaminophen to provide relief. Remember that some fever can be beneficial in fighting illness (see "Fever" section), so don't treat more often than necessary.

FOR CONGESTION / RUNNY NOSE

As a general principle, we prefer that you use nasal saline drops or spray (Ocean®, Nasal®, or generic equivalent) to irrigate the nostrils and clear mucous and to do so **only if the mucous is bothersome to your child.** If the saline is not effective and the excess drainage is making your child uncomfortable, you may use an oral decongestant. Please note that in general **we strongly discourage the use of oral decongestants** and prefer either spray decongestants or integrated therapies. You may refer to the sections on "Colds" and "Integrated Management of Respiratory Illnesses" for further guidance.

OVER-THE-COUNTER (OTC) MEDICATION RECOMMENDATIONS AND DOSAGES

ORAL DECONGESTANTS

AGE / WEIGHT	Dimetapp®, Benadryl® Syrup	Sudafed®, Pediacare®, Triaminic ® Syrup	Dimetapp® Drops, Pediacare® Drops
6-12 mos. / 14-18 lbs.	1/2 tsp.	1/4 tsp.	0.8 ml.
1-2 yrs. / 19 - 24 lbs.	3/4 - 1 tsp.	1/2 tsp.	1.2 ml.
2-3 yrs. / 25 - 36 lbs.	1 - 1 1/2 tsp.	1/2 - 3/4 tsp.	1.6 ml.
3-6 yrs. / 37 - 48 lbs.	1 1/2 tsp.	3/4 -1 tsp.	-
6-8 yrs. /49 - 60 lbs.	2 tsp.	1 tsp.	-

These medications may be given every 4 to 6 hours (CHECK INDIVIDUAL PRODUCT INSTRUCTIONS TO CONFIRM). They may be given with antibiotics. If the product does not already contain ibuprofen or acetaminophen, you may also give those medications as directed in the table for that section. These preparations are intended for the relief of discomfort but may cause irritability, agitation, restlessness, or lethargy and sedation in some children. If you note these symptoms in your child, discontinue the medication and avoid its use in the future.

An alternative treatment option that results in minimal side effects compared to oral medication is the use of NASAL SPRAY DECONGESTANTS. (Note: Extended use of nasal decongestants may cause a persistent runny nose. For that reason, **limit their use to 5 to 7 DAYS ONLY.**)

SPRAY DECONGESTANTS

AGE	Neosynephrine 1/8% (0.125 solution)	Neosynephrine 1/4% (0.25 solution)	Afrin® (0.025 solution)	Afrin® (0.05 solution)
12 - 24 mo.	1 drop every 4-6 hours	-	-	-
2 - 5 yrs.	2-3 drops every 4-6 hours	1 drop every 4-6 hours	1-3 drops every 12 hours	-
5 - 12 yrs.	-	2-3 drops every 4-6 hours	-	2-3 sprays every 12 hours
> 12 yrs.	-	same as above	-	same as above

OVER-THE-COUNTER (OTC) MEDICATION RECOMMENDATIONS AND DOSAGES

FOR COUGH

Please refer to the "Cough" section for discussion of specific treatment measures. If your child is unable to rest because of the cough, you may treat with:

AGE/ WEIGHT	Delsym® Dose every 12 hours	Robitussin DM®, Vick's 44® (or other 10 mg dextro-methorphan /5ml syrup) Dose every 6 hours	Robitussin® Pediatricdrops Dose every 4-6 hours
6-12 mos./14-18 lbs.	¹/₄ tsp	¹/₂ tsp	1.25 ml
12-24 mos./19-24 lbs.	¹/₂ tsp	³/₄ tsp	2.5 ml
2-3 yrs./25-36 lbs.	³/₄ tsp	1 - 1¹/₂ tsp	2.5 ml
3-5 yrs./37-48 lbs.	1 tsp	1¹/₂ - 2 tsp	-
5-10 yrs./49-72 lbs.	1 - 1¹/₂ tsp	2 tsp	-
>10 yrs./>72 lbs.	1¹/₂ - 2 tsp	2 - 3 tsp	-

These recommended doses are FOR PRODUCTS WHICH CONTAIN ONLY DEXTRO-METHORPHAN. **Do not use the above chart for dosing combination products such as Tylenol Sinus®, etc.** Dextromethorphan may be given along with antibiotics, decongestants, antihistamines, natural products, and any other "multi-system relief" product that does **NOT** already contain dextromethorphan. (**NOTE: In general, we do not recommend the use of multi-drug formulations** as their use may lead to under- or over-dosage for your child's symptoms.)

FOR ITCHING DUE TO HIVES, CHICKEN-POX, ECZEMA, ALLERGIC REACTION, ETC.

Benadryl® or generic diphenhydramine may be used every 4 to 6 hours. **Do not exceed 6 doses per day.** This medication often causes mild drowsiness. If your child experiences agitation, discontinue its use. Weight is the most accurate method to determine the dose for your child. **NOTE: DO NOT put Caladryl® lotion or any other diphenhydramine-containing lotion or cream on your child's skin WHILE administering this oral medication.** This can lead to over-dosage from the oral and skin absorption of the medication.

15

OVER-THE-COUNTER (OTC) MEDICATION RECOMMENDATIONS AND DOSAGES

BENADRYL®/diphenhydramine dosage

AGE/ WEIGHT	Liquid 12.5mg/5ml	Chewable 12.5 mg	Tab/cap 12.5 mg	Tab/cap 25 mg
6-12 mos. 12-21 lbs.	$^1/_2$ tsp.	-	-	-
12-18 mos. 22-35lbs	1 tsp.	-	-	-
18 mos. - 4 yrs. 36-47 lbs.	$1^1/_2$ tsp.	$1^1/_2$	-	-
4 - 8 yrs. 48 - 65 lbs.	$2 - 2^1/_2$ tsp.	$2 - 2^1/_2$	2	1
8-12 yrs. 66 - 87 lbs.	$3 - 3^1/_2$ tsp.	$3 - 3^1/_2$	3	1
> 12 yrs. 88 lbs. +	4 tsp.	3 - 4	3-4	1 -2

FOR HAYFEVER / ALLERGY SYMPTOMS

For acute allergy reactions, Benadryl® or generic diphenhydramine is recommended in the doses above. Non-sedating relief is now available without a prescription with loratadine (for example, Claritin®). Loratadine is dosed ONCE every 24 hours as follows:

AGE	loratadine syrup (5 mg./tsp.)	tablet 10 mg	loratadine +decongestant (e.g., Claritin-D 24®)
2-5 yrs.	1 tsp.	$^1/_2$	-
6-11 yrs.	2 tsp	1	-
12 and older	-	1	1

FOR EAR PAIN

In addition to using acetaminophen and/or ibuprofen (see previous tables for dosages), there are other measures that can help relieve your child's ear pain. If there are no surgically inserted pressure equalization tubes in your child's eardrums, and no bloody or pus discharge from the ear canal, you may instill drops for pain relief into the ear canal. Sweet or olive oil, Willow Garlic

Oil™, or Auralgan® (a prescription pain reliever) may be used as follows: Place 3 to 4 drops in the affected ear canal. Place a slightly moistened portion of a cotton ball at the entrance of the canal to help retain the oil inside. **This should be repeated as often as every 15 to 20 minutes until pain is relieved and then as often as necessary after that. For a more soothing effect, these oils may be gently warmed before each use. TEST THE WARMED OIL FIRST on your skin to be sure it's not too hot.**

FOR SORE THROAT PAIN

See "Throat" section for a discussion of methods for relieving throat pain associated with any illness.

FOR VOMITING

See "Vomiting" section for discussion of oral rehydration and instructions for the use of Emetrol®.

FOR MOTION SICKNESS

For the prevention of motion sickness, the following medications may be used. Because these medications may be sedating, we recommend use only in the child known to be prone to vomiting with motion sickness.

AGE	DRAMAMINE® /dimenhydrinate May dose every 6-8 hours		BONINE® /meclizine May dose ONCE every 24 hours	
	12.5 mg/ 4 ml syrup	50 mg tablet	12.5 mg tablet	25 mg tablet
2-5 yrs.	3/4 - 1 1/2 tsp	1/4 - 1/2 tab	1	1/2
5-12 yrs.	1 1/2 - 3 tsp	1/2 - 1 tab	2 - 4	1 - 2

FOR DIARRHEA

In general, we recommend **DIETARY CHANGES FIRST** rather than medication to treat diarrhea. Please refer to the "Diarrhea" section for dietary management and guidance regarding if and when to medicate your child with Imodium® AD. When using Imodium® AD, it should be given once, then repeated as directed below **only** if two or more episodes of diarrhea follow that initial dose.

AGE /WEIGHT	IMODIUM A-D® /loperamide		
	1 mg /5 ml liquid	2 mg tablet	2 mg caplet
less than 1 yr.	NOT RECOMMENDED	-	-
1-2 yrs. /20-26 lbs	³/₄ - 1 tsp	¹/₂ tab	-
2-5 yrs. /26-40 lbs	1 tsp	¹/₂ tab up to 3X /day	-
6-8 yrs. /40-60 lbs	2 tsp	1 tab up to 2X /day	1 cap up to 2X /day
8-12 yrs. /60lbs +	2 tsp	1 tab up to 3X /day	1 cap up to 3X /day

ADMINISTERING INTEGRATED TREATMENTS

This section is dedicated to helping you **develop the confidence and the skills to use the many easy, safe, and effective integrated therapies** outlined in this reference handbook. In this section you will find instructions on how to use each of the major therapies, dosing guidelines for nutrient supplements, and other topics. To ensure optimal effectiveness, please read the area applicable to the alternative therapy that you are interested in before you begin to use that therapy.

AROMATHERAPY

Aromatherapy relies on the administration of essential oils to affect the therapeutic response. Aromatherapy is very safe in children, provided the essential oil used is **"therapeutic grade."** Information regarding the grade should be available where you purchase the oils. As with any therapeutic method in children, aromatherapy has the potential for very powerful stimulation and thus, for safety reasons, we recommend you **use essential oils under the guidance of a qualified health-care professional.** We have intentionally kept **essential oils** use very simple in this reference handbook. With this small, select list of essential oils known to be safe and effective, we believe you will be able to accomplish significant relief.

Often, there is more than one species of a particular plant from which essential oils are derived for therapeutic use. In this case it is **very important to be certain you are using the specific species that has been recommended.** For example, a commonly used essential oil, eucalyptus, has at least eight different species, but we **specifically** recommend eucalyptus radiata.

There are four ways to administer essential oils for aromatherapy:

1. Massage. The first is to make massage oil by adding 4 to 6 drops of the essential oil into 1 ounce of a "carrier oil" (for example, almond, avocado, apricot kernel, olive, jojoba, or hazelnut oil) and mix well. This may then be used as massage oil. By applying it to the skin of your child, the essential oil is absorbed through the skin and into the system, where it can have its therapeutic effect. This technique is especially good if the oil is massaged into the soles of the feet. To check for skin sensitivity, apply a small amount of massage oil to a small area of normal skin and watch for approximately 1 hour. If no reaction occurs, you may comfortably use it as a massage oil.

2. Bath. You may add 2 to 5 drops of essential oil to a bath of warm water and let your child soak for a comfortable period of time.

3. Skin Wash. You may use essential oils as a skin wash. To make an essential oil skin wash, add 5 to 6 drops of the oil to 1 ounce of purified water and shake vigorously. You may apply it to the skin with a cotton pad or from a spray bottle 2 to 3 times a day.

4. Steam Inhalation. Heat 2 quarts of purified or bottled water just before a boil and then remove from the heat. Place it in a pan or bowl on a counter or chair where your child can easily lean over the pan. When you are ready to actually do the steaming, **test the temperature of the steam yourself** and if it seems comfortable, show your child how near to the steam to place his face for comfort and safety. Young children may be most comfortable on your lap. With his head in the proper position, place 2 to 3 drops of the essential oil in the water and drape a towel over his head and the pan. Instruct your child to breathe deeply for several minutes and stay close by to ensure the safety and effectiveness of the treatment. (Note: Always monitor your child closely to prevent accidental spills or burns.)

   If your child has a **cold or sinus infection, encourage him to breathe through his nose. If he has a cough, encourage him to breathe through his mouth. (NOTE: If he has asthma, first test his comfort with steam only, and if he does not have difficulty with the steam, then you may add the essential oils with close observation. If his wheezing or coughing increases you should discontinue the treatment immediately.)**

If you would like to have essential oils on hand, the most frequently used oils in our reference handbook are Eucalyptus radiata, Ravensara aromatica, Roman Chamomile, Lavender, and Mandarin. "Therapeutic grade" can be purchased in specialty stores that carry such oils.

HERBAL REMEDIES

Herbal remedies are prepared in a variety of ways for administration. Herbs intended for internal use can be found as loose herbs for infusion tea, tea bags for beverage tea, tinctures, glycerites, syrups, capsules, and tablets. As topical agents they can be found as salves, creams, and gels. Herbs are available both as single herb remedies and as combinations of herbs designed to accomplish a common therapeutic effect (for example, decrease congestion).

Herbs are derived from plants that are generally safe for ingestion; therefore, teas, tinctures, glycerites, syrups, capsules, and tablets can be added to food or beverages for safe, easy, and effective administration. However, **they should be respected as having therapeutic potency and should be administered in strict accordance with the dosing guidelines found on the product package.** (Note: If your child develops rash, wheezing, or other allergic symptoms while taking herbal remedies, discontinue use and contact your health-care provider for advice.)

Herbal teas are readily available and are one of the mainstays of traditional herbal medicine around the world. For therapeutic purposes it is important to distinguish between non-medicinal beverage teas (teas made from tea bags) vs. a properly prepared infusion of the loose herbs. While beverage strength herbal teas are a wonderful way for children to enjoy natural teas—and they certainly may have an effect—**only teas prepared as infusions of loose herbs are considered to have enough potency to have a genuine therapeutic effect.** Herbal teas can be very effective and easy to administer to children.

To **prepare an infusion of herbal tea:** Begin by bringing 1 cup of water to a boil, turn off the heat, add 1 teaspoon to 1 tablespoon of the herb (leaf, flower, and/or root). Cover and let plant material steep in the recently boiled water for 10 to 20 minutes. To make an herbal tea more palatable to a child, prepare the tea in half organic apple juice and half water. By freezing the juice-based tea, you can make "popsicles" out of teas. **Dosage, of course, varies according to age and weight and potency of the tea.** The table below outlines general dosing guidelines thought to be safe and effective; follow them unless your health-care provider has given you more specific guidelines.

AGE	AMOUNT OF TEA	FREQUENCY
1 to 2 years	$^1/_4$ cup	3 times a day
2 to 6 years	$^1/_2$ cup	3 – 4 times a day
6 to 11 years	$^3/_4$ cup	3 – 4 times a day
12 years and up	1 cup	3 – 4 times a day

Liquid extracts are concentrated extracts of the herb or herbs, obtained by soaking the herb in a liquid extractant. From a therapeutic point of view liquid extracts **are the most potent way to administer an herbal remedy. A tincture is a liquid extract in which alcohol is used as the extractant.** Tinctures have a very strong and frequently bad taste. They may also contain significant amounts of alcohol. These traits make them less favorable for use in younger children. **A glycerite is a liquid extract in which glycerine, a sweet-tasting material derived from vegetable oil, is used as the extractant.**

Because glycerites are far better tasting and free of alcohol, they are a much better therapeutic choice for children.

Syrups are compounds containing the herbal remedy and a large amount of thick sweetener such as honey, molasses, or sugar. They are mainly used for herbal cough and colds preparations.

Capsules and tablets are convenient methods of administering herbs but they have two limitations. First, they are the least potent of the methods available for administering herbs. Second, they are not an option for children who are unable to swallow them.

Herbal remedies (for example, Calendula extract) that are prepared as topical agents (that is, salves, creams, or gels) can be used safely when applied directly to the skin according to the dosing guidelines on the package. In the unlikely event that your child appears to react to the topical preparation, it should be discontinued and you should notify your health-care provider.

On some occasions, for example before surgery, we may recommend avoiding a particular herb, so be sure to discuss their use with your health-care provider.

HOMEOPATHIC REMEDIES

Homeopathic remedies are produced as **"classic" remedies**, which contain only one remedy and in only one strength (potency), or as **"complex" remedies**, which are formulas that contain several different remedies in multiple potencies. Classic remedies are used in such specific circumstances (for example, a specific type of "flu" in a specific type of person) that they generally require great expertise to prescribe and are beyond the scope of this handbook. The **complex formulas are designed to treat a disease complex** (for example, a specific remedy for sinus infections) and thus are well-suited to our style of integrated medicine. We have selected them as our primary way to use homeopathic remedies.

Homeopathic remedies come in a variety of forms for administration. For internal use they are most commonly found as tablets, drops, and globules (pellet-sized tablets). For external or topical use they can be found as creams, ointments, and gels.

Homeopathic remedies can be very effective in treating a wide variety of illnesses. Because homeopathic remedies are highly diluted substances, they have great safety but this also makes them very delicate. **In order for them to be effective, they must be carefully handled and administered according to the following simple guidelines:**

- Homeopathic remedies are absorbed through the membranes of the mouth; therefore, **they must be placed in the mouth at a time when the mouth is clean of food and drink.** The remedies should be given when the **child has not had any food or drink for at least 15 minutes. After the final remedy is given, the child should not eat or drink for at least another 10 to 15 minutes.** In infants this time can be reduced to 5 minutes if absolutely necessary.

- Homeopathic tablets **should not be touched with your hands.** You may tap the tablets or globules out of the bottle and into the lid and then into the child's mouth. They may then be chewed but not swallowed. Allow the remedy to dissolve in your child's mouth. For younger children the tablet may be tapped onto a spoon and then crushed between two spoons into a powder. The powder may then be placed directly into the child's mouth or may be mixed with bottled water and then placed into the mouth.

- **Homeopathic drops are preserved in grain alcohol and thus may have a stinging taste to them.** If this taste does not bother your child, drops may be put directly into the mouth. Another option is to dilute the drops with bottled water and then place them in the mouth. Ideally, neither the hands nor mouth should touch the dropper as this could neutralize the remaining remedy in the bottle.

- When administering more than one homeopathic remedy for an illness, **do not place them in the mouth at the same time.** Each individual remedy, whether tablets or drops, should be **administered separately and spaced approximately 5 to 10 minutes apart.**

- **When dosing remedies several times in one day, the dosing intervals do not need to be evenly spaced.** For example, if you are scheduled for three doses in one day it is just as effective to give a dose at 8 a.m., 6 p.m., and 9 p.m. as it is to space them evenly throughout the day. This eliminates the need to have the remedies given at school or at daycare. You should administer them in whatever way is most convenient for your schedule. The doses should, however, be spaced at least 1 hour apart.

- **The dose of a homeopathic remedy is usually 1 tablet; 3 to 4 globules; or 4 to 8 drops per dose.** But if a larger amount is given, it is safe and no adjustments need to be made in the treatment plan. The only significant way to alter the dosing administration of a homeopathic remedy is to change how often it is given. For chronic problems **(for example, chronic constipation) or mild illnesses (for example, a mild cold) the normal frequency of administration is 2 to 3 times per day. For more intense illnesses (for example, influenza or asthma) the dosing frequency** should be 5 to 6 times per day initially, and then when things begin to improve, the frequency can be reduced to 2 to 3 times per day. The duration of treatment depends mostly on the illness being treated. In general, the treatment should last several days beyond the resolution of the illness.

BACH FLOWER REMEDIES

While Bach Flower Remedies are not produced in the exact same way as most homeopathic remedies, for practical purposes they can be considered as homeopathic remedies. Thus, the dosing guidelines are the same as described above in "HOMEOPATHIC REMEDIES."

DIET AND NUTRITIONAL SUPPLEMENTATION

Good nutrition is the cornerstone of good health, and it is not only critical to eat a healthy and nutritionally balanced diet for health maintenance, but dietary changes and nutritional supplements can promote restoration and maintenance of good health. Some basic principles of nutritional support in illness are recommended in the specific sections of this handbook with the dosing guidelines provided below.

In general, whenever your child is suffering from a respiratory illness, it is wise to reduce or eliminate milk, all dairy products, and all citrus fruit and their beverages (for example, orange and grapefruit). These foods tend to cause an increase in respiratory mucous production, which is counter-productive when the body already has too much mucous in the respiratory system. Other dietary changes specific to a given illness may be found within that illness section itself.

It is also a very good idea to increase your child's fluid intake to maintain good hydration as well as keep the respiratory mucous thin and easily flowing. The best beverage is water or other clear liquids (Pedialyte® and $^1/_2$ strength Gatorade® are preferred to fruit juices). The following table is a safe guideline for administering fluids for good hydration.

AGE	OUNCES OF WATER PER DAY
2 to 5 years old	12 to 18 ounces
5 to 12 years old	18 to 24 ounces
12 Years and up	32 to 48 ounces

Nutritional supplements can play a significant role in helping children through illnesses. These potential benefits could be in the form of preventing illness, support for or resolution of an active illness, and recuperation from an illness. Nutritional recommendations have been made in the individual illness section (where applicable) with the intent that dosing guidelines will be found in this section. Each specific nutritional supplement recommendation will be found below with a brief discussion of its usefulness.

VITAMIN A

Vitamin A is a required nutrient in multiple aspects of the immune system and is therefore essential to healthy function of the immune system. It is also a critical nutrient for the repair and maintenance of the cells of mucosal surfaces (that is, the surfaces that line the entire respiratory tract). These two aspects of vitamin A make it an important nutrient to use as a supplement to support children with respiratory illnesses, especially infections. **Vitamin A may be given once daily for 1 to 2 weeks** using the dosing guidelines as follows:

AGE	MAXIMUM DAILY DOSE GIVEN ONCE A DAY
1 to 3 years	2,000 IU
3 to 6 years	2,500 IU
6 to 10 years	3,500 IU
11 and up	4,000 IU

VITAMIN C

The use of vitamin C to prevent colds and minimize cold symptoms is still controversial; however, we do recommend it. Vitamin C is safe and generally well-accepted by children. Our experience suggests that many children clearly benefit, while others do not. **You must judge for yourself the impact of vitamin C on your own child.** Vitamin C may also improve the speed of a child's recovery from a respiratory infection and thus may be useful for several weeks after the initial infection. The vitamin C doses that we recommend during a cold are as follows:

AGE	DOSE
6 months to 2 years	100 mg 3 – 4 times daily
2 years to 5 years	250 mg 3 – 4 times daily
5 years to 10 years	500 mg 3 – 4 times daily
10 years and older	1000 mg 3 – 4 times daily

VITAMIN E

Vitamin E is often used topically to soothe damaged skin and promote healing. For topical use vitamin E is easily obtained from gel caps, which are designed for oral administration. Puncture the gel cap with a safety pin and squeeze out the vitamin E oil into the palm of your hand. Then gently rub a small amount of the oil into the irritated or damaged skin once or twice daily until the skin appears healed.

Vitamin E can also help the body heal from inflammation (for example, from infections) and can be taken internally. Using the dosing guidelines below, **give your child vitamin E orally until the healing process appears to be complete.**

AGE	DOSE
2 to 4 years	10 IU 2 – 3 times daily
4 to 7 years	20 IU 2 – 3 times daily
7 to 12 years	30 IU 2 – 3 times daily
12 and older	50-75 IU 2 – 3 times daily

ZINC

Zinc is one of the most important nutrients supporting the function of the immune system; as such, zinc supplementation may benefit the immune response at the onset of a respiratory infection. **Zinc may also possess a direct inhibitory effect on an invading virus,** enhancing **the immune system's** ability to help fend off respiratory infections. Zinc comes in a variety of products and is safe for children when used in strict accordance with dosing and administration guidelines found on the product package.

Homeopathic preparations of zinc are available and may be used according to the instructions on the package insert.

ADMINISTERING INTEGRATED TREATMENTS

Zinc also comes in the form of a lollypop or sucker on a stick (for example, Zinc Pops), suitable for children 6 months or older. Again, follow the dosing guidelines on the package insert.

There are also numerous brands of zinc lozenges (and suckers for younger children) suitable for anyone old enough to safely suck a hard candy. **It is recommended that you follow the dosing guidelines on the product you are using. NOTE: Many of these products contain other herbs (for example, echinacea) and nutrient supplements (for example, vitamin C). These ingredients should be considered part of the total daily dose of those particular supplements, to avoid the risk of overdose.**

Zinc is **most effective when taken as early in the illness as possible and then continued for 2 to 5 days.** However, zinc supplementation should not be taken for more than 7 days because it can lose its effectiveness and there is more chance for intolerance with prolonged use. For dosing zinc suckers and lozenges, always follow the package guidelines. If there are no guidelines, you may safely follow the guidelines below.

AGE	MAXIMUM DAILY DOSE (for a maximum of 7 days)
6 to 12 months	6 mg
1 to 2 years	10 mg
2 to 12 years	10 mg
12 and up	15 mg

MAGNESIUM

Magnesium supports many metabolic functions in the body. As a dietary supplement it enhances the absorption and metabolism of calcium and vitamin C. **In some children it will improve their bowel movements.** If the recommended doses do not achieve the desired effect, you may want to call your health-care provider for more specific recommendations.

AGE	DOSE
1 to 3 years	100-150 mg once daily
3 to 6 years	150-200 mg once daily
6 to 11 years	200-300 mg once daily
11 years and up	300-400 mg once daily

EFAs (Essential Fatty Acids)

Essential fatty acids (EFAs) are fats that we obtain primarily from our diet. They support a wide variety of different functions in the body and are widely believed to help keep skin healthy, support and develop nervous system function, and support the immune system. Our diets are often lacking in adequate amounts of EFAs, so it is a good idea to take a supplement. There are many good supplements—for example, primrose oil, borage oil, and black currant oil—but one of the most balanced, inexpensive, and best-tasting EFA supplements is **flaxseed oil.** General dosing guidelines are as follows:

AGE	DOSE
6 to 12 months	$1/4$ tsp. twice daily
1 to 3 years	$1/2$ tsp. twice daily
3 to 6 years	1 tsp. twice daily
6 to 12 years	2 tsp. twice daily
12 and up	3 tsp. twice daily

PROBIOTICS

Probiotics refers to the use of supplements to the diet that replace or encourage the **development of favorable bacteria in the colon (large intestine).** These favorable bacteria are essential to our good health. They support normal digestion, produce nutrients, improve elimination, and support a healthy immune system. There are many factors that can upset the normal balance of these favorable bacteria, including exposure to antibiotics both as medicines and in our foods, other chemicals in our diet, gastrointestinal infections, and a variety of other stresses.

Acidophilus is a common species of favorable bacteria in humans, and the name is often used to refer in a generic way to the "probiotic" concept. Acidophilus is the species of bacteria used to convert milk into yogurt. However, yogurt does not contain enough acidophilus to significantly affect the make-up of bacteria in the colon. To increase the number of favorable bacteria in the colon (which is especially important after the use of a prescription antibiotic), a probiotic supplement must be used.

Probiotic supplements contain different species of bacteria because as we grow and develop, the species of bacteria in our colon changes. Thus, **we recommend that you use a probiotic supplement that is specific to your child's age.** Information regarding the age-appropriate probiotic and its dosage is usually available on the product label.

It is best if you use a probiotic that is stable in food so that you can administer it in food. If the supplement is not stable in food, it should be taken on an empty stomach. Powders, liquids, tablets, and capsules are all effective, and you should select the delivery form most convenient to your child. We generally recommend using the supplement twice daily for 3 to 6 weeks (unless otherwise specified by this reference handbook or your health-care provider).

While dietary changes are not necessary when using probiotics, the effectiveness of probiotics may be enhanced by simple dietary changes, such as reducing or eliminating red meat, dairy products, and refined sugar.

At the end of each illness section there is an "Integrated Therapies" guide that suggests specific herbs that may benefit in the healing process of that illness. There is a very large selection of natural care products that may accomplish the same therapeutic goals, and it is beyond the scope of this handbook to cover them all. This list is designed to provide an easy starting place to find products that we believe are safe and effective. You may substitute products that you also know to be safe and effective and have the same therapeutic goals.

GENERAL SUPPORT
1. Valerian root: Herbs For Kids—Valerian Super Calm™
2. Echinacea/Astragalus: Herbs For Kids—Echinacea/Astragalus™ (NOTE: Because echinacea is an immune stimulant, we do not recommend its use in diseases in which the immune system is overactive, such as asthma or eczema.)

PAIN
1. Willow bark extract: Herbs For Kids—Willow Garlic Oil™
2. For sore throat: Traditional Medicinals Teas—Throat Coat™

RESPIRATORY
1. Horehound: Herbs For Kids—Horehound Blend™
2. Cherry bark: Herbs For Kids—Cherry Bark Blend™

DIGESTIVE
1. Ginger: Herbs For Kids—Minty Ginger™
2. Mint: Herbs For Kids—Minty Ginger™
3. Carob Powder: May be purchased as a food product at most natural food stores.

SKIN
1. Tea tree oil: A variety of good brands are available.
2. Aloe vera: A variety of good brands are available.
3. Calendula cream: We recommend Weleda brand or any of a variety of good brands that are available.

Note that any of these products can be found in most health food stores; in the event that your local store doesn't carry them, or there is no health food store in your area, they can all be readily purchased on the internet.

BLENDED TEAS
1. For relaxation: Sleepy Time Tea™
2. For sore throat and cough: Throat Coat™

HOMEOPATHIC REMEDIES LIST

At the end of each illness section there is an "Integrated Therapies" guide that suggests specific homeopathic remedies that may benefit in the healing process of that illness. There is a very large selection of natural care products that may accomplish the same therapeutic goals, and it is beyond the scope of this reference to cover them all. **This list is designed to provide an easy starting place to find products that we believe are safe and effective. You may substitute products that you also know to be safe and effective and have the same therapeutic goals.**

GENERAL SUPPORT

1. Heel Engystol®
2. BHI Inflammation®
3. Heel Gripp-Heel®
4. Heel Traumeel® (drops or tablets)
5. Heel Belladonna-Homaccord™ or Belladonna 6X or 30X potency
6. BHI Exhaustion®
7. BHI Lightheaded®

PAIN

1. BHI Spasm-Pain® or Heel Spascupreel®
2. Heel Viburcol Drops®
3. BHI Headache®
4. Hyland's Teething Tablets®

RESPIRATORY (Ear, Nose, Throat, Sinus and Lungs)

1. BHI Bronchitis®
2. BHI Asthma®
3. Heel Euphorbium Drops® or Euphorbium Sinus Relief Nasal Spray®
4. BHI Cold®
5. BHI Eye®
6. Heel Traumeel Pure Eye Drops®
7. BHI Allergy®
8. BHI Cough®
9. BHI Chamomilla Complex®
10. BHI Sinus®
11. BHI Hayfever Nasal Spray® or Heel Luffeel Nasal Spray®

DIGESTIVE

1. BHI Chamomilla Complex® or Hyland's Colic Tablets™
2. BHI Constipation®
3. BHI Diarrhea®
4. BHI Nausea®

SKIN

1. Heel Traumeel Cream®
2. BHI Skin®
3. Heel Apis-Homaccord® or Apis 6X potency

URINARY

1. BHI Uri-Control®

Note that any of these products can be found in most health food stores; in the event that your local store doesn't carry them, or there is no health food store in your area, they can all be readily purchased on the internet.

FIRST-AID PROCEDURES
FOR COMMON EMERGENCIES AND INJURIES

An important part of parenting is preparation for an emergency. This brief review contains very general information about childhood emergencies and injuries and what to do should they occur. **We strongly encourage you to take a first-aid class at a nearby hospital or through the Red Cross. Practical, hands-on experience through a certified class will give you the added confidence to initiate all first-aid procedures and, in the event of an emergency, will likely save a child's life! There is no substitute!**

Accidents are the leading cause of injury and death in children and can be prevented to a large degree with attention to your child's environment. **Every home should have a well-stocked first-aid kit that includes basic supplies and medications.** Store your kit in a safe place. Keep it updated and remember to bring a kit with you when you are away. We recommend that your kit include the following:

SUPPLIES:
Ace bandage
Adhesive bandages
Bulb syringe
Cotton pads
Rubbing alcohol and/or hydrogen peroxide
    for disinfecting wounds and sterilizing supplies
Scissors with round tips
Sterile gauze pads
Tape
Thermometer
Tweezers

CONVENTIONAL MEDICINES:
Antiseptic ointment (such as Neosporin® or Bacitracin®)
Acetaminophen (Tylenol®) and ibuprofen (Advil®) in an age-appropriate
    concentration (i.e., infant/children's, etc.) for pain and fever management
Calamine lotion
Diphenhydramine (Benadryl®) for allergic reactions
Emetrol to quiet vomiting
$1/8$% Neosynephrine (Pediatric Afrin® or Little Noses®)

FIRST-AID PROCEDURES
FOR COMMON EMERGENCIES AND INJURIES

HERBAL REMEDIES:
Aloe vera gel
Calendula cream
Minty Ginger™ (Herbs for Kids) for upset stomachs

HOMEOPATHIC REMEDIES:
Apis Hommacord® (BHI)
Traumeel® (BHI) ointment and tablets

BACH FLOWER REMEDIES:
Rescue Remedy™

NUTRITIONAL SUPPLEMENTS:
Oral rehydration supplies (such as Pedialyte®, etc.)

A good book on the application of general first-aid procedures is recommended. In addition, you should post the following important information and phone numbers prominently:

- Emergency: 911
- Poison Control Center:
- Fire Department:
- Police:
- Ambulance:
- Parent Work Number:
- Pediatrician:
- Hospitals:
- Neighbor/Close Friend:
- Pharmacy:

It is strongly recommended that all parents and caregivers take a certified course in cardiopulmonary resuscitation (CPR). The Red Cross and local hospitals provide these courses. Your ability to intervene in the event of an emergency can save the life of a child.

FIRST-AID PROCEDURES
FOR COMMON EMERGENCIES AND INJURIES

WHEN A CHILD STOPS BREATHING:

1. Shout for help: "Call 911."
2. Then, clear your child's mouth of possible foreign objects—see "Choking" section.
3. Straighten the airway by placing the nose even with the middle of the chest.
4. Begin mouth-to-mouth breathing. Your child will most likely resume breathing very quickly. If not, continue your efforts until help arrives.

WHEN A CHILD IS CHOKING:

Although your child may appear to be choking, his airway may not be obstructed. If he can speak, cry, or cough, his airway is not obstructed and he is not choking. Allow him to clear his airway with your supportive assistance. True signs of choking include inability to vocalize, drooling, and panic. Your child may turn blue and become unconscious. Call 911 while you initiate the following:

For infants under 1 year old:

1. Lay infant face down across your lap or forearm while supporting his head at a level lower than his chest.
2. Give five quick, firm blows high on the back between the shoulder blades.
3. If that doesn't clear the airway, turn your child face up, keep head low, press two fingertips below baby's nipples, and give five upward thrusts.
4. Alternate between back and chest maneuvers until either the infant begins breathing again or loses consciousness.

If the infant loses consciousness, lay him on a flat surface.

1. Check the mouth for any visible objects. Remove with your fingers any objects you can see. DO NOT BLINDLY ATTEMPT TO DISLODGE AN OBJECT.
2. Tip his head back and gently lift the angle of the jaw. Begin mouth-to-mouth resuscitation by covering the infant's mouth and nose with your own mouth.
3. Administer 2 gentle breaths of air. If the chest does not move, repeat 5 back blows and 5 chest thrusts and check the infant's mouth again for any foreign bodies. Attempt mouth-to-mouth resuscitation again.

35

For children over 1 year of age:

1. Stand behind your child; place your fist with thumb knuckle against the middle of your child's chest at the low edge of the ribs.

2. Give four quick upward thrusts; repeat until your child expels the foreign body or loses consciousness.

If the **child loses consciousness,** lay him on a flat surface and call 911.

1. Check the mouth for any visible objects. Remove with your fingers any objects you can see. DO NOT BLINDLY ATTEMPT TO DISLODGE AN OBJECT.

2. Tip his head back and gently lift the angle of the jaw.

3. Begin mouth-to-mouth resuscitation by pinching his nostrils closed, covering his mouth with yours and giving 2 slow rescue breaths. If his chest wall moves, begin CPR.

4. If his chest does not move, the airway is still obstructed. Straddle your child and place your stacked hands on your child's abdomen below the rib cage. Give 5 quick, upward thrusts to force the obstructing object out of the windpipe.

5. Repeat steps 1 through 4 until breathing is restored or help arrives.

BITES: ANIMAL AND HUMAN

Any bite that breaks the skin requires immediate attention. If a bite wound causes uncontrollable bleeding, call 911 immediately. If the bleeding does not stop after 10 minutes of direct pressure or if the wound is split open or gaping, call your health-care provider for instructions on appropriate care. Otherwise, begin cleansing the wound vigorously with soap and water for 10 minutes while you contact your health-care provider for further directions. Scrub the wound enough to make it re-bleed a little.

If a snake has bitten your child, seek immediate medical attention by calling Poison Control!

Both animals' and humans' mouths contain bacteria that are injected into the wound, incurring a higher risk of infection than other injuries. Bite wounds are tetanus prone; if your child has not had a tetanus booster within the past 5 years, a booster will be recommended.

If a wild animal has bitten your child, try to contain the animal so it can be tested for rabies.

Support your child's immune system and wound healing with the following supplements:

– Apply antibiotic ointment to the wound as directed by a health-care provider.

– Traumeel® 1 tablet dissolved in mouth 4 to 6 times/day for 10 to 14 days.

BITES AND STINGS: INSECT

If your child is experiencing difficulty breathing, call 911 immediately. If your child has a history of severe reactions/allergies to insect stings, have an emergency sting kit ("EpiPen®") available and know how to use it. Take it on all trips and family outings. They are available by prescription only.

Look for signs of a severe reaction: excessive pain and swelling, hives, extreme lethargy, difficulty breathing. If this is so, call your health-care provider immediately. Your child will probably need to visit an emergency room.

To remove a tick, grab the tick firmly right next to the skin where it is attached (you may use a tissue to grab it). Turn the entire body of the tick counter-clockwise several turns until it comes free in your fingers. Using this method will usually result in the whole tick coming free, including the mouth. You may also use tweezers to grasp the tick as close to the skin as possible. Pull back slowly and firmly until the tick is released. Wash, rinse, and disinfect your hands and the area of the bite immediately. Apply an antibiotic ointment. Call your health-care provider if you cannot remove the tick's head or if you notice an unusual rash or illness within the first several days following a tick bite.

With bee or wasp stings, remove the stinger, if possible, by gently scraping it out (for example, with the edge of a credit card). Then, thoroughly wash and rinse the area. Do not squeeze the wound. For painful stings, apply ice immediately; then apply a paste of meat tenderizer (or baking soda) and water. This paste may be applied for the next 24 hours. Use acetaminophen or ibuprofen for pain relief.

For itching, use oral Benadryl® elixir. See "OTC Drug Recommendations and Dosages" section. Calamine lotion applied topically 4 or 5 times daily will also reduce itching. For severe itching, apply 1% hydrocortisone cream (over-the-counter) two to four times a day. For fast relief, apply firm, sharp pressure using a fingernail to the bite for 10 seconds. Aloe vera gel or Calendula (cream or gel) can provide relief from itch and irritation also.

A sting or insect bite may cause a localized skin infection some hours or days after the bite. If you see redness and/or yellow discharge from the wound, apply antibiotic ointment 4 times per day. Call your health-care provider if you see an area of spreading redness or red streaks around the bite.

Bite prevention:

Insect repellants containing DEET (N,N –diethyl-m-toluamide) are the most effective products available to prevent illnesses induced by mosquito and tick bites. In 2003, the American Academy of Pediatrics advised that over-the-counter insect repellants containing up to 30% DEET can be safely recommended for children 2 months of age and older when applied as directed. DEET-containing products are NOT for use in infants less than 2 months of age. You should select the product concentration of DEET for the desired length of protection level, presuming once daily application.

5% DEET gives duration of protection of about 1.5 hours.

10% DEET gives duration of protection of about 2 to 4 hours.

20% and greater DEET lasts for longer than 4 hours, etc.

DEET should be applied to clothing, shoes, and exposed skin, taking care to avoid your child's hands, mouth, eyes, and open cuts or wounds. Be sure to remove all DEET-treated clothing and wash all DEET-exposed skin with soap and water upon returning inside. Clothes treated with DEET should be laundered first before wearing them again. We do not advise the use of "combined" DEET and sunscreen products, because the temptation to re-apply this product, as one would with sunscreen alone, could lead to excess DEET exposure. Always refer to the directions on the product label when using any insect repellant.

BURNS

Steam or hot liquids, hot ovens or stoves, hair and clothing irons, heating grates and cigarettes are the most common causes of burns. Lye, acids, or other caustic substances are common causes of chemical burns. Burn injuries can be described by their severity:

First-degree Burns: These burns are the least severe. With a first-degree burn, the skin is red and painful, but blisters are not present and the skin is not broken. Sunburn, burns from brief contact with hot objects, chemical burns, and steam exposure typically cause first-degree injury. First-degree burns usually improve within two days. Most first-degree burns will respond to the same treatments used for sunburns. Please refer to the section titled "Sunburns" for more information.

Second-degree Burns: Second-degree burns cause injury to the deeper layers of the skin. They produce swelling, pain, and blisters. Severe sunburn or burns from hot liquids frequently cause second-degree burns. These burns may take 2 to 3 weeks to heal.

Third-degree Burns: Third-degree burns involve all layers of the skin and the burned area can appear white, yellow, black, or deep red. Pain is minimal because nerve endings are damaged. Burns that result from direct fire contact, prolonged contact with hot substances and electrical burns can cause a third-degree burn. If the burn area is larger than a quarter, a skin graft may be recommended to prevent severe scarring.

Burn injuries can also be described by the amount of skin involved. For example, in children, the surface area of the hand correlates with approximately 1% of the body surface area.

Home Care

1. Immediately immerse the burned area in cool water for 5 to 15 minutes. Clothing can be removed after thorough rinsing; however, you should not remove clothing if you suspect a third-degree burn. Gently pat dry and inspect the severity of the burn. If it is a chemical burn, remove clothing before rinsing.

2. Electrical burns can be interrupted by removing the electrical current (that is, turning the switch or breaker off). Never touch a person while he is being electrically shocked. If you cannot turn the current off, use a nonconductive item (such as a wooden broom handle) to remove the source of current away from the child. Any child who has received an electrical burn needs immediate medical attention, even if the damage appears minor.

3. All presumed second- and third-degree burns and burns to the hands and face should be reported immediately. If there are extensive areas of second- (more than 20% of the body surface area) or any third-degree burns, your child will need immediate medical attention. Your health-care provider may be able to treat less serious burns in their office with special cleansing and antibiotic creams. However, serious burns to the face or hands are referred to the hospital burn units.

4. Do not apply butter, oil, grease, or creams. These substances can trap heat and worsen the injury. Do not pop blisters.

5. First-degree burns can be treated at home with aloe vera pulp, gel, or liquid. Apply gently three times daily and lightly cover with either gauze or a bandage. Acetaminophen or ibuprofen may help with discomfort (see "OTC Drug Recommendations and Dosages" section).

6. Rescue Remedy™ can be used to help with anxiety and fear. Place 2 to 3 drops on your child's tongue or place in a half glass of water to sip. This may be repeated every 5 to 10 minutes until he is calm.

FIRST-AID PROCEDURES
FOR COMMON EMERGENCIES AND INJURIES

CUTS AND ABRASIONS

The main goals in treating cuts and abrasions are to stop the bleeding, prevent infection, and promote healing.

1. Stop the bleeding by applying pressure with a clean cloth or gauze for up to 5 to 10 minutes. You may place ice on the cut to decrease bleeding. If your child has a cut in the mouth, an ice pop may help.

2. Once the bleeding has stopped, rinse the wound with generous amounts of cool water. Remove any dirt or foreign matter from the cut by flushing with running water. Gently clean the wound with mild soap and water for at least 5 minutes.

3. Apply antibiotic ointment (Neosporin® or Bacitracin®). Calendula cream or ointment may be applied to superficial wounds as they heal. (Note: Neosporin Plus® has a pain reliever included to offer more rapid relief.)

4. Cover the wound with a dressing (for example, a Band-Aid®).

5. Clean the wound and reapply an ointment and dressing once daily until the wound has healed.

6. Call for further medical assistance if:
   - the bleeding does not stop within 10 to 15 minutes of applying pressure.
   - the wound edges are gaping. (Call promptly—within 2 to 4 hours —if you think your child may need stitches.)
   - the wound appears deep or extensive.
   - there is still debris in the wound after 15 minutes of scrubbing.
   - a deep wound involves the mouth, face, or hand.
   - the wound appears infected or has not healed after 10 days.

7. A tetanus booster is indicated if your child has not received a booster in the past 5 years or has not been completely vaccinated. It can be given within 24 hours of the injury.

8. Rescue Remedy™ may be administered to help calm a distressed child. Place 2 to 3 drops on your child's tongue or place in a half glass of water to sip. This may be repeated every 5 to 10 minutes until he is calm.

HEAD INJURY—See "Head Injury" section.

FIRST-AID PROCEDURES
FOR COMMON EMERGENCIES AND INJURIES

POISONING

Your local Poison and Drug Center specializes in up-to-date information on all kinds of poisonings and ingestions and how to treat them.

When you call the Poison and Drug Center, please have the following important information available:

1. Name of substance and its ingredients. The bottle label is essential.
2. Time of ingestion, if known.
3. Amount of ingestion, if known.
4. Amount of ingested substance remaining in bottle.
5. Age and weight of child.
6. If any vomiting has occurred, do you see pills, etc., in the vomit?
7. Associated symptoms, such as coughing, vomiting, drowsiness, agitation, or other behavior changes.

TRAUMA—Bone, Muscle, Ligament, and Joint

Any traumatic injury can be scary for both you and your child. Remain calm and reassure your child.
For any injury, the following therapies can be helpful:

- Rescue Remedy™ may be administered to help calm a distressed child. Place 2 to 3 drops on your child's tongue or place in a half glass of water to sip. This may be repeated every 5 to 10 minutes until he is calm.
- Traumeel® cream or ointment can be administered to assist rapid healing. It can be applied 4 times per day to any injury in which the skin is intact. This can be applied for 10 to 14 days or until injury resolves.
- Traumeel® tablets can be given 4 times per day orally if the skin is damaged. This can be administered for 10 to 14 days or until the injury resolves.

Sprains are often associated with a twisting injury and commonly occur in the knee, ankle, wrist, and shoulder. Usually they are minor injuries caused by stretching or superficial tearing of ligaments around the joint.

Minor sprains can be treated as follows:

1. Ice should be applied immediately for up to 30 minutes to reduce swelling. You may continue ice application for 15 minutes every hour for the first four hours. Continue ice application every 2 to 3 hours through the second day.

2. Wrap an elastic bandage around the joint to minimize swelling and reduce movement (for at least the first 48 hours). The bandage should be "snug" but not "tight." Numbness, tingling, or increased pain indicate the bandage is too tight.

3. Elevate the affected limb while your child is awake. At night, prop the injured area up with an extra pillow.

4. Support with a splint, sling, or crutches may be necessary to restrict movement and reduce weight bearing. After the first 24 hours, activity that does not cause pain can be encouraged.

5. Give Motrin® or Advil® (ibuprofen) as an anti-inflammatory and pain reliever. (Please see "OTC Medications and Recommendations" section for dosing guidelines.)

6. Call your health-care provider if:
   - there is significant pain and swelling, especially within 30 minutes following the injury.
   - the child cannot move the joint or extremity.

Strains are associated with strenuous use of a muscle, often occurring after long hikes and competitive sports.

1. Massage sore muscles with ice for 30 minutes. Repeat 3 to 4 times during the first day. If pain persists after the second day, apply a warm compress or have your child soak in a warm bath for 10 minutes 3 to 4 times/day until pain resolves.

2. Give ibuprofen every 6 to 8 hours for the first 2 days.

3. Call your health-care provider if:
   - there is significant pain or swelling.
   - pain and swelling lasts longer than 3 days.

Bruised Muscles or Bones often occur when an extremity is struck by an object (such as a football) or kicked. (Follow directions above for "Strains.")

1. Rest the injured part as much as possible.

2. Anticipate improvement within the first 48 hours, and complete resolution of discomfort within the next 14 days.

3. Call your health-care provider if the pain is severe or the swelling is increasing after the initial injury has stabilized.

Fractures

Bone fractures can be very painful, produce considerable swelling, and reduce normal movement of the affected area. If the pain or swelling is severe, the extremity cannot be moved, the extremity appears deformed, or the trauma itself was considerable (bad fall, crushing injury, bone has broken through the skin), your child may have fractured a bone.

If you suspect your child has a broken bone:

1. DO NOT MOVE HIM! Try to immobilize that extremity with a home-made splint. If unable to do so, call 911.

2. Initial treatment is the same as for sprains (see previous section).

3. Call your health-care provider for further directions. Treatment will likely be handled in an emergency room or orthopedist's office.

4. After the fracture has been acutely managed (i.e., with splinting or casting), the following supplements can facilitate healing:

   • Calcium (250 mg) and magnesium (125 mg) given two times/day for 2 months.

   • Vitamin C once per day for 2 months dosed as follows:
     under 2 years, 100 mg
     2 - 10 years, 250 mg
     10 - 18 years, 500 mg

   • Feed your child a diet rich in lean protein, calcium (green leafy vegetables and low-fat dairy products) and vitamin D (enriched dairy products and eggs).

   • Avoid sodas, which deplete calcium from bones.

   • Traumeel® is a homeopathic remedy designed to speed the body's recovery from injury. It may help to minimize swelling and inflammation. It may be taken (1 tablet or 4 drops per dose) 3 to 6 times a day until the healing is complete.

TRAUMA, TOOTH

When a permanent tooth has been knocked out, quick treatment and proper care of the tooth are critical. Handle the tooth by the top (crown), not the root.

1. Rinse the tooth with cold water—DO NOT CLEAN.
2. Try to reset the tooth back in the socket. Call your dentist for further instructions.
3. If you are unable to reset the tooth, put it in a cup of milk or water, and then call your dentist immediately for instructions.

If a damaged permanent tooth is loose, leave it alone and call your dentist during office hours. If a "baby tooth" is knocked out, stop the bleeding for now and call your dentist during office hours. There is no need to reset a baby tooth if it is knocked out.

Description/Physiology

Abdominal pain is a common symptom that accompanies many childhood illnesses. There are several very different triggers for abdominal pain. Some causes are obvious and straightforward while others remain complex and difficult to diagnose. There are both acute and chronic forms of abdominal pain.

It is beyond the scope of our book to detail every cause and every expected course, so this section will depart from the handbook's usual format to serve more as a directory of causes. Because causes of abdominal pain are so varied, this section will guide you to other sections in the handbook that may help more clearly pinpoint the exact cause.

We are most concerned about differentiating between serious triggers (medical or surgical emergencies) versus common triggers that can be managed at home (stress-induced or viral infections).

Causes/Epidemiology

Abdominal pain may result from pain generated in any organ or structure in the abdomen and some adjacent areas. Thus, there may be abnormalities with the stomach and intestines, the liver, the spleen, the gallbladder, the pancreas, the kidneys, any of the supporting soft tissue structures, the bladder, the ovaries, the uterus, and so forth. There may also be pain from adjacent organs, such as the lungs and the bones of the pelvis and spine.

Abdominal pain may be caused by infection, trauma, obstruction, constipation, colic, emotional upset, food allergies, menstrual cramps, motion sickness, and urinary tract infections, to name just a few.

Expected Course

The anticipated course of abdominal pain depends largely on its trigger and to a lesser extent on the age of the child and the child's general health. Pain ranges from very mild, such as with overeating or indigestion, to severe and unbearable, such as with appendicitis or the passage of a kidney stone. Abdominal pain may be acute in its onset or chronic in nature.

Abdominal pain rarely occurs by itself. There are usually accompanying symptoms, such as fever, vomiting and/or nausea, diarrhea, sore throat, "flu"-like symptoms, etc.

We recommend that you look at your child's entire health and symptom profile. This full picture helps your health-care provider best decide what the trigger is, assess its severity, predict its typical course, and ultimately craft the proper treatment.

If the abdominal pain is chronic or recurrent, it is always wise to create a diary of the abdominal pain and its accompanying symptoms. Include in your diary any of the following details:

- Description of the pain:
  - Time of day of pain.
  - Exact location of pain.
  - Duration of the pain episodes.
  - What the pain keeps your child from doing (for example, walking, school, etc.).
  - What makes the pain worse?
  - What makes the pain better?
  - All associated symptoms.
  - Obvious triggers of pain.
- Describe bowel habits and any recent changes.
- Is there any blood in the stool?
- Does your child also have a sore throat?

Your very careful documentation of your child's history, along with your health-care provider's examination and occasional labs tests, will likely identify the cause. If your health-care provider needs additional help in making the correct diagnosis, they may ask for an evaluation with a pediatric gastrointestinal specialist.

We recommend that you now read any of the sections in this book relevant to your child's current illness. The symptoms most associated with abdominal pain and discussed in detail in this book are:

- Constipation
- Dehydration
- Diarrhea
- Fever
- First Aid—Poisoning
- Headaches
- Infectious Mono
- Influenza
- Stress
- Throat
- Vomiting

Home Care

Home care recommendations focus first on recognizing and assessing your child's entire health picture. In general, treatments that target specific symptoms (such as vomiting and diarrhea) may reduce the abdominal pain that is also part of that illness.

Primary goals are to relieve immediate abdominal pain and discomfort, carefully observe your child and document all symptoms, respond to significant worsening of pain, and, in some instances, remove or avoid the causative agent.

Please read this entire section and all other relevant sections to develop a home approach that best fits your child's particular situation. Several common treatment themes emerge for early relief of abdominal pain.

1. Rest. Keep your child quiet and reduce activity as much as possible.

2. A warm water bottle or beanbag can be gently placed on the abdomen, allowing the weight to soothe abdominal pain.

3. Offer your child only clear liquids and avoid dairy products until the course of symptoms and the source of the abdominal pain become more evident.

4. See if your child will have a bowel movement.

5. Stop all prescription medications for several hours. If you have been giving ibuprofen, stop that also.

6. Document all symptoms in a diary detailed as above.

7. Stay calm and provide comfort and reassurance.

 ## Integrated Therapies

(Please refer to the section on "Administering Integrated Treatments" on page 19 for guidance on using any of the therapies that follow.)

AROMATHERAPY

• An aromatherapy bath or massage with the essential oil lavender can soothe and relax your child's anxiety and restlessness when in pain. Add 2 to 5 drops of oil to a warm bath and allow your child to soak for a comfortable period of time.

HERBAL REMEDIES (For quick reference please refer to the "Herbal Remedies List" on page 31 and the inside cover.)

- Ginger is a valuable herb that may be helpful in quieting down an "upset stomach" and decreasing abdominal cramping. For dosing, follow the package labeling accurately.
- Mint can also soothe an upset stomach. Mint teas, lightly sweetened, have the added benefit of being an excellent way to get fluids into your child. Mint tinctures are also available. For dosing, follow the package labeling accurately.
- Chamomile may also soothe abdominal cramps. Chamomile tea, lightly sweetened, has the added benefit of being an excellent way of getting extra fluids into your child.

HOMEOPATHIC REMEDIES (For quick reference please refer to the "Homeopathic Remedies List" on page 32 and the inside cover.)

- A homeopathic remedy designed to have a soothing effect on abdominal cramping may be useful. It can be given hourly (or more often if directed by your health-care provider) as needed for relief of cramping until the pain is relieved. (Pain 1)
- A homeopathic remedy designed to ease intestinal colic or cramping symptoms may be useful. It can be given hourly (or more often if directed by your health-care provider) as needed for relief of cramping until the pain is relieved. (Digestive 1)

BACH FLOWER REMEDIES

- Rescue Remedy™ may be of use if your child is uncomfortable from the illness, stress, or anxiety. You may use 2 drops every 10 minutes to every few hours to calm restlessness as needed.
- A lukewarm bath with 10 drops of Rescue Remedy™ added to the bathwater is often very effective at relieving agitation and stress in general.

NUTRITIONALS AND SUPPLEMENTS

- Probiotics

DIETARY GUIDELINES

- Your child may not feel well enough to eat, so don't force him. Instead, make sure that he continues a good intake of fluids and drinks extra water to ensure good hydration. You may use the following table as a general guideline for water in addition to normal fluid intake:

AGE	OUNCES OF WATER PER DAY
2 to 5 years old	12 to 18 ounces
5 to 12 years old	18 to 24 ounces
13 and up	32 to 48 ounces

 ## When to Call Your Health-care Provider

Call immediately if:
- The pain is unbearable and your child cannot be consoled.
- There is blood in the stool. (See "Diarrhea" or "Constipation" sections.)
- Your child vomits blood. (See "Vomiting" section.)
- Your child becomes progressively more lethargic or difficult to arouse.
- The pain is especially severe in the right lower part of the abdomen.
- Your child has rapid and labored breathing.
- There is significant back pain.
- Your child has significant pain with urination or abnormalities of urine flow. (See "Urinary Tract Infection" section.)
- There has been trauma to the abdomen and pain worsens.
- Your child vomits repeatedly and meets criteria for dehydration. (See "Vomiting" and "Dehydration" sections.)
- Your child loses consciousness because of the pain.

Call within 24 hours if:
- Your child has steadily worsening abdominal pain.
- There are signs of worsening dehydration.
- There appears to be a chronic pattern of abdominal pain emerging.

 ## Other Relevant Sections

Colic
Constipation
Dehydration
Diarrhea
Fever

ABDOMINAL PAIN

First Aid—Poisoning
Headaches
Infectious Mono
Influenza
Throat
Stress
Urinary Tract Infection
Vomiting

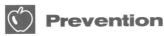 **Prevention**

Please refer to the appropriate sections that discuss symptoms associated with abdominal pain.

Description/Physiology

Asthma is a chronic inflammatory disease of the airways characterized by difficulty breathing, and the most common symptom is wheezing. The child and parents can often recognize a wheeze as a whistling sound produced while breathing out. Children often describe a sensation of "chest tightness," especially while breathing in. In a younger child, asthma often presents with a persistent cough and a prolongation of exhalation. Asthma has had many names over the years, such as "reactive airways disease," but the most recent terminology defines asthma by the frequency of wheezing and severity of the symptoms.

Inflammation of the airways, a primary feature of asthma, is caused by an overactive response of the immune system to triggers such as viral respiratory infections, allergies, the stress of exercise, and inhaled irritants (such as cigarette smoke). Another feature of asthma is airway hyper-reactivity, which means the muscles surrounding the airways in the lungs are more likely to spasm and narrow in response to a stimulus (such as an infection or allergen). The third feature of asthma is increased mucous production in response to the same stimuli. When inflammation, reactivity, and increased mucous production are combined, the airway becomes very narrow, and air can no longer pass with ease. Thus, a child will wheeze as air enters and escapes through these narrowed passages.

Causes/Epidemiology

Asthma is one of the most common chronic diseases of childhood, affecting millions of children each year. It is often inherited, but it may be seen in children with no family history. "Atopy" is a word used to describe a predisposition to respond to allergens such as pollens, spores, and other substances in the environment. Atopic children have a stronger risk for developing asthma and often have a history of eczema and seasonal allergies. Children with asthma may have a history of recurrent bronchiolitis early in life (see "Bronchiolitis" section). Asthma is more frequently diagnosed in school-age children due to the natural progression of the disease, an increased awareness of symptoms, and the improved ability of child and parent to describe symptoms. Asthma is occasionally diagnosed in younger children (less than 3 years old) who present with chronic cough, recurrent wheezing, and/or allergies.

Asthma exacerbations may be caused by exposure to one of the following triggers:

- viral respiratory infections
- bacterial infections of the sinuses, ears, and lungs
- inhaled allergens from plants (weeds, grasses, and trees), animals, and molds
- inhaled irritants such as tobacco smoke, paint fumes, smoke from burning wood, air pollution, dust, and perfumes
- exercise, especially in cold or dry air
- gastro-esophageal reflux (regurgitation)

 ## Expected Course

An asthma exacerbation typically resolves when the trigger is removed and the inflammation has subsided. The duration depends on what triggered the episode, the severity of the child's asthma, and the type of and response to the interventions that are used. Though it is a chronic disease, many children grow out of their asthmatic tendencies. Current medical research indicates that longstanding/untreated inflammation of the airways may lead to permanent changes of the tissue and resultant diminished breathing capacity.

 ## Contagiousness/Immunity

Asthma itself is not contagious.

 ## Home Care

Once your child has been diagnosed with asthma you will receive many tools for identifying and treating exacerbations at home. Your health-care provider may give you an "asthma action plan" to help you adjust treatment as symptoms change. Home care can be best utilized in combination with ongoing check-ups with your health-care provider.

Principles of home management of asthma involve prevention of exposure to triggers and rapid identification and treatment of exacerbations.

1. Early identification of exacerbations:
   Take note of the early warnings or signs of an asthma attack.
   - Does your child cough or feel short of breath with exertion or conversation?

- Is your child developing a cold?
- Has your child been exposed to a known trigger?
- Has your child been coughing more at night or in the morning?

A peak flow meter can be used to detect increasing obstruction in the airways. Please talk to your health-care provider about obtaining one.

Early treatment of an exacerbation can prevent a more severe episode with the associated fearful, sleepless nights, and even hospitalization. If you note worsening of symptoms, please follow the instructions on your asthma action plan or call your health-care provider promptly for further guidance.

2. Treatment of exacerbations

Your health-care provider will direct the medical treatment of an asthma exacerbation.

The following medications are commonly used to treat asthma and target the underlying abnormality. All of these medications are available by prescription only. Your health-care provider, or your asthma specialist, will provide instructions for their use based on the age of your child, the severity of symptoms, and triggers.

Begin treatment early, as many children wheeze soon after they develop coughs or colds. Start the asthma medicine, inhaler, or nebulizer at the first sign of any coughing or wheezing. Remember that the best "cough medicine" for your child with asthma is the asthma medicine itself. Always keep this medicine handy. Take it with you on trips. If your supply runs low, obtain a refill.

A. Airway constriction is reversed by medications that dilate the bronchial tubes, such as albuterol and levalbuterol (Xopenex®). These medicines reduce symptoms (cough, shortness of breath, wheezing) by relaxing tightened muscles surrounding the airway, thereby increasing the movement of air. These medications can be stimulating, causing increased heart rate, hyperactivity, and anxiousness. Albuterol and levalbuterol (Xopenex®) can be given through a nebulizer (an aerosolized mist treatment). Albuterol can also be given through an inhaler (also called an MDI or "puffer"). An inhaler is most effective when used with a special chamber called a spacer. The primary role these medications play is to "rescue" a child from an acute flare-up of his asthma. They play a less significant role in maintenance or preventive therapy, although "pretreatment" before exercise or exposure to a known trigger will help avoid asthma symptoms.

B. Airway inflammation is treated by anti-inflammatory medications.

Steroids are often used to calm the overactive immune system's response to a trigger by reducing the swelling in the airways. Inhaled steroids, by nebulizer or inhaler, are a mainstay in the treatment and prevention of asthma. Oral steroids are occasionally used in severe exacerbations to provide fast and significant relief from restricted airways.

Non-steroid oral medications such as Singulair® block the inflammatory effect of a group of substances that are released from cells in the lungs in response to a trigger event. Singulair® is taken every day, even when the child is asymptomatic, in order to provide maximal protection.

Finally, inhaled medications such as Intal® can prevent cells from releasing inflammatory substances. Be sure to discuss with your health-care provider the choice, frequency, and duration of treatment with any of these preventive medications.

C. General supportive measures for an asthma exacerbation.

Remember, during an asthma exacerbation your child will feel "stressed," not only by the illness itself but possibly from the medication used to treat the illness. Provide a calm environment. Do not allow visitors and turn off the telephone. Play one of your child's favorite movies or soothing music.

Good fluid intake helps keep the normal lung mucous from thickening. Loose mucous is more easily coughed out of the airway. Clear fluids are best. Sipping warm fluids may reduce wheezing, as well.

Humidifiers in dry climates can generally be helpful in all respiratory diseases. However, in asthma your child's response to a humidifier may vary, and some children feel worse with increased humidity. Thus, humidifiers must be used on a trial-and-error basis. See what works best for your child.

Your child may go to school during mild asthma attacks but should avoid physical education class on those days. Arrange to have the asthma medicines available at school. It is also important to advise the school about your child's current condition. If your child uses an inhaler and is responsible enough to participate in a treatment plan, he should be permitted to keep it with him so that he can use it readily. Participation in sports or active play may need to be postponed until symptoms have subsided.

Integrated Therapies

(Please refer to the section on "Administering Integrated Treatments" on page 19 for guidance on using any of the therapies that follow.)

AROMATHERAPY

- Aromatherapy with either eucalyptus radiata or ravensara aromatica, combined with mandarin may soothe the symptoms of asthma during an attack. They may also decrease the frequency of asthma attacks when used as part of a preventive strategy. You may make a preparation by adding 2 to 3 drops of each essential oil to 1 ounce of carrier oil. Then massage into the soles of your child's feet. You may also administer them by steam inhalation or a bath. In general it is best to avoid other aromatherapies during the treatment of asthma.

HERBAL REMEDIES (For quick reference please refer to the "Herbal Remedies List" on page 31 and the inside cover.)

- NOTE: Because echinacea is an immune stimulant, we do not recommend its use in diseases in which the immune system is overactive, such as asthma or eczema.
- Horehound may be very effective in reducing mucous production and improving a wet cough. It may help in the recuperative phase of asthma if there is a significant amount of mucous production. For dosing, follow the package labeling accurately.
- Valerian root is a mild herbal sedative that may offer some help in easing a child with a significant cough. Valerian root may be most useful at bedtime. For dosing, follow the package labeling accurately.
- Mullein leaf as an infusion tea may also help decrease the frequency of asthma attacks when used as part of a preventive strategy. Use two cups daily for 3 to 6 months.

HOMEOPATHIC REMEDIES (For quick reference please refer to the "Homeopathic Remedies List" on page 32 and the inside cover.)

- A homeopathic remedy designed to resolve bronchial irritation and coughs (manifesting as a deep chest cough), especially those associated with an asthma exacerbation, may be useful. The remedy can be taken 2 to 3 times daily during the acute illness and continued for up to 1 to 4 weeks after, as indicated by the persistence of the cough. (Respiratory 1)

- A homeopathic remedy designed to reduce bronchial spasm and wheezing, especially if associated with an asthma exacerbation, may be useful. The remedy can be taken 2 to 3 times daily during the acute illness and continued for up to 1 to 4 weeks after, as indicated by the persistence of the cough. (Respiratory 2)
- A homeopathic remedy designed to support the defense system during viral infections may be useful. It can be taken 3 to 6 times daily when the virus is active (for example, fever, lethargy, etc.). (General Support 1)
- A homeopathic remedy designed to decrease inflammation and fever from infections may help prevent deterioration and shorten the recovery time. It can be taken 3 to 6 times daily when the virus is active (for example, fever, lethargy, etc.). (General Support 2)

BACH FLOWER REMEDIES

- Rescue Remedy™ may be of use if your child has anxiety with episodes of coughing. You may use 2 drops every 10 minutes to every few hours as needed to calm restlessness.
- A lukewarm bath with 10 drops of Rescue Remedy™ added to the bathwater is often very effective at relieving agitation and stress in general.

NUTRITIONALS AND SUPPLEMENTS

- Vitamin A
- Vitamin C
- Vitamin E
- EFAs

DIETARY GUIDELINES

- It is best to avoid all dairy products and citrus fruits because they may increase or thicken respiratory mucous.
- Warm foods such as soups, warm cooked grains (for example, oatmeal), and teas should be given.
- Cold foods, foods high in sugar, and fried foods should be avoided.
- Your child may not feel well enough to eat, so don't force food. Instead, make sure he continues a good intake of fluids. He should drink extra water to ensure good hydration. You may use the following table as a general guideline for water in addition to normal fluid intake:

AGE	OUNCES OF WATER PER DAY
2 to 5 years old	12 to 18 ounces
5 to 12 years old	18 to 24 ounces
13 and up	32 to 48 ounces

INTEGRATIVE SUPPORTIVE CARE

- Please read the section "Integrated Management of Respiratory Illnesses."

 # When to Call Your Health-care Provider

Call immediately if:

- There is shortness of breath or rapid breathing rate (over 60 breaths per minute in an infant or over 40 breaths per minute in children over the age of 2 years), especially in the absence of fever.
- Your child is struggling for each breath.
- Your child is making grunting noises with each breath.
- Your child is unable to speak or cry or sleep because of difficulty breathing.
- Your child's lips are blue.
- Your child's wheezing began suddenly after ingesting a medication or food, or being stung by an insect.
- You are instructed to do so by your asthma action plan (that is, the peak flow readings are not improving, despite intervention).

Call within 24 hours if:

- You suspect your child is having his first asthma attack.
- Your child has had severe attacks in the past and is developing symptoms again.
- You need refills on any asthma medications.
- You would like to have an asthma action plan that includes some type of breathing assessment, such as a peak flow meter.
- You would like to talk about stress reduction techniques for your asthmatic child.
- Your child is having symptoms with exercise only.

Other Relevant Sections

Bronchiolitis

Colds

Eczema

Hay Fever

Integrated Management of Respiratory Illnesses

 Prevention

Early prevention can start in infancy by minimizing a child's exposure to tobacco smoke (please begin during pregnancy!). In addition, breast-feeding may also reduce your child's risk of atopy (allergic disease).

To reduce or eliminate exposure to allergens:

- If pets are a trigger, please consider finding a new, loving home for your pet. If this is not possible, keep the pet out of your child's bedroom/play rooms and filter any air ducts in those rooms.
- Dust mites are a common trigger. Anticipate potential exacerbations in humid places (greater than 50% humidity). Likewise, cockroach dander can also cause significant problems.
- To avoid exposure to pollens and outdoor molds, stay inside with the windows closed during seasons that are the most problematic. Pollen counts are usually higher in the afternoon. Air conditioning is preferable to evaporative cooling. Allergy treatments can help enhance lifestyle (see "Hay Fever" section) by allowing more liberal exposure to the outdoors.
- Vacuum carpets 1 to 2 times per week. Use a HEPA filter or double bag in the vacuum. Consider replacing carpet with vinyl, tile, or wood flooring.
- Use only properly cleaned humidifiers and take note if humidifier use increases your child's symptoms.
- Use of air filtration systems or HEPA room air purifiers can be helpful, as can regular duct cleaning.

Yearly influenza vaccination is strongly recommended for all asthma patients.

Regular exercise can improve lung function in asthmatics. Some children may need medication (such as albuterol) prior to exercise to prevent exercise-induced symptoms.

Relaxation and breathing techniques are invaluable in preventing and supporting an asthma exacerbation. Consider enrolling your child in yoga classes or other techniques that foster relaxation. Biofeedback and guided imagery can also be helpful. A 20-minute massage performed by parents at bedtime has been shown to improve lung function in asthmatics. The bottom line: Help your child learn to relax before and during an asthma exacerbation!

Evaluate your child's stress level. Is he overbooked? Overwhelmed? Helping him manage stress (please see the "Stress" section) will not only help his asthma now, but will prepare him for the future.

ATHLETE'S FOOT (TINEA PEDIS)

 ## Description/Physiology

Athlete's foot is typically a red, scaly, cracked, itchy, raw or burning rash between the toes and sometimes on the soles of the feet. The rash may ooze a clear substance when scratched. It may burn, sting, and develop into sores.

 ## Causes/Epidemiology

Athlete's foot is a fungal (yeast) infection that grows well on the warm, damp skin of the feet. It is often the result of wearing shoes that trap moisture and prevent air flow, such as tennis shoes. It is most commonly seen in adolescents.

 ## Expected Course

With proper treatment, athlete's foot usually clears within two to three weeks. It can recur several times in the same season.

 ## Contagiousness/Immunity

Athlete's foot is minimally contagious. The fungus will not grow on normal, dry skin. Your child may continue sports activities and school PE. It is a commonly held view that athlete's foot can be acquired in locker rooms, swimming pools, etc. This is rarely true. Do wash your hands carefully after you apply medication, however.

 ## Home Care

1. Anti-fungal cream. You may use Tinactin® or Micatin® or Lotrimin® lotion or cream, all available over-the-counter (OTC). Spray forms are also effective. First, rinse your child's feet in clear water and dry the feet carefully (especially between the toes). Then, apply a thin layer of the anti-fungal cream twice daily directly to the rash and beyond the rash borders. Continue using the anti-fungal cream until the rash has cleared and then for 5 additional days.

   When the infection is particularly inflamed, we may recommend a combination anti-fungal cream and a mild anti-inflammatory cream such as Cortaid® (1/2% hydrocortisone). On rare occasions your health-care provider may use a prescription medication.

2. Dryness. Athlete's foot improves more rapidly if feet are kept dry. The cure is accelerated if your child goes barefoot or wears sandals or flip-flops as much as possible. Avoid non-porous leather shoes and rubber-soled shoes. Only cotton socks should be used and socks should be changed daily. Dry your child's feet carefully after baths, showers, and swimming. Teach your child to do so routinely after water exposure.

3. Scratching. Discourage scratching as much as possible, as this will delay the cure and may spread the infection. A dose of Benadryl® may be necessary to reduce significant scratching.

4. Foot odor. With the above treatment, foot odor will often improve as the athlete's foot resolves. There is rarely a need to treat the odor. If foot odor continues, it is possible that shoes are now the problem, so wash the tennis shoes twice to purge them of the fungus and the odor, or replace them.

 Integrated Therapies

(Please refer to the section on "Administering Integrated Treatments" on page 19 for guidance on using any of the therapies that follow.)

HERBAL REMEDIES (For quick reference please refer to the "Herbal Remedies List" on page 31 and the inside cover.)

- Tea tree oil, for topical use only, has a natural antibiotic and antifungal effect. It can be used to treat or prevent athlete's foot. If the skin appears to become infected, use the tea tree oil 2 to 3 times a day, or as a preventive 2 to 3 times a week. A tea tree oil skin wash, gel, or cream is best, as the full-strength oil may be too strong for your child's skin.

- Aloe vera or calendula applied topically can reduce itching and soothe irritated skin. They are available in gel, lotion, or cream. For dosing, follow the package labeling accurately.

HOMEOPATHIC REMEDIES (For quick reference please refer to the "Homeopathic Remedies List" on page 32 and the inside cover.)

- A homeopathic cream designed to soothe inflamed or irritated skin may be useful. It can be applied directly to the infected area 3 times a day. (Skin 1)

NUTRITIONALS (only required for chronic recurrent infections)
- Vitamin A
- Vitamin E
- EFAs
- Probiotics

 ## When to Call Your Health-care Provider

Athlete's foot is not an emergency. Your call and treatment can usually wait until the next morning.

Call immediately if:
- The rash is a painful, red, hot rash spreading away from the toes.

Call within 24 hours if:
- The athlete's foot is not improved in one week with the above treatments.
- It is not completely cured after using the above treatments for two weeks.
- It starts to look infected and pus starts draining from the rash.

 ## Prevention

- Teach and/or keep your child's feet as dry as possible.
- Encourage your child to wear only dry socks. Shoes worn over damp socks enhance the moist, fungus-growing environment.

 ## Other Relevant Sections

Eczema
Impetigo

Description/Physiology

Bronchiolitis is an inflammation of the smallest airways of the lungs, the bronchioles.

Bronchiolitis is characterized by some or all of the following symptoms:

- Wheezing a high-pitched, whistling sound produced during breathing out (expiration).
- Rapid breathing with a significant increase in your child's normal respiratory rate. For example, if your infant normally breathes 20 times per minute, he might breathe with an increased rate of 60 breaths per minute.
- Tight breathing (your child has to push the air out).
- Coughing with an often harsh quality and often with sticky mucous.
- Early respiratory symptoms often include fever and runny nose.
- Symptoms similar to asthma.
- Overall increased work of breathing with deeper excursions of the chest wall with breathing—that is, chest heaves up and down more.

Causes/Epidemiology

Bronchiolitis can be caused by a number of respiratory viruses, and the best known and most common of these is the Respiratory Syncytial Virus (RSV). RSV has become a household name and is generally associated with the most severe form of bronchiolitis. Bronchiolitis occurs most often in children who are less than 2 years old.

Bronchiolitis occurs every winter and accounts for about one-half of many hospitals' admissions. Whereas infants and toddlers with RSV and other viruses may develop full-blown bronchiolitis, older children and adolescents with the same virus may simply develop cold symptoms without the wheezing component. Each child responds differently according to his own anatomy and immune system.

Once a first bout of bronchiolitis has occurred, your child may be more prone to future episodes. Allergies may also play a role in triggering bronchiolitis. These recurrent bouts of bronchiolitis may continue each year for 3 to 4 years after the initial case.

The wheezing of bronchiolitis is caused by a narrowing of the smallest airways in the lung (bronchioles). This narrowing results from inflammation and swelling of the lining of the airway, mucous production, and mucous entrapment in these airways.

 ## Expected Course

The initial symptoms of bronchiolitis are typical cold symptoms such as runny nose, cough, and fever, followed by a worsening phase during which time wheezing may develop. The wheezing itself may last several days, while the other cold symptoms may last up to a week. The cough itself may linger up to 4 to 6 weeks. See "Cough" section.

Your child will likely drink less and sleep restlessly. He may be agitated and fretful. Decreased interest in drinking may lead to varying degrees of dehydration, which further thickens mucous and slows healing. See "Dehydration" section. The sleep-deprived child is always slower to recover.

There are relatively few later complications of bronchiolitis. Bacterial pneumonia, bronchitis, and sinusitis are uncommon complications. Most of the serious problems are the result of worsening wheezing and cough, which may lead to an oxygen requirement, dehydration, and even hospitalization.

Only a small percentage of children with bronchiolitis require hospitalization. Hospitalization may involve treatment with oxygen, intravenous fluids, a nebulizer, respiratory therapy, and, rarely, steroids. Evaluation of your wheezing child may include measuring oxygen levels, obtaining a chest x-ray, doing a nasal wash for RSV, and assessing hydration. The sickest children are sent to the emergency room for further evaluation and treatment, but many of these children will be released from the ER with careful instructions for home management and follow-up. Others may be admitted to the hospital.

The diagnosis of asthma may be considered after 2 or 3 such wheezing bouts. There is always a fine line between the diagnosis of asthma and recurrent bronchiolitis. In general, if your child continues to wheeze with every viral infection, he has asthma. However, labeling a child as "asthmatic" may carry with it an emotional charge, so we must look carefully at the history and evaluate factors such as age, frequency, family history, and triggering events such as viruses and allergies before this diagnosis is made. Issues about asthma require a thorough discussion, both to understand the disease processes better and to properly develop a plan tailored to your child's particular needs. See "Asthma" section.

Contagiousness/Immunity

The viruses that cause bronchiolitis are found in nasal and oral secretions. They are spread by sneezing or coughing (airborne) or by hand-to-nose or hand-to-eye or hand-to-mouth contact. Children do not develop permanent immunity to RSV or to any other respiratory virus that causes bronchiolitis. Thus, the same child can acquire RSV several times, although not likely more than once in the same season.

The lingering cough of bronchiolitis is not generally contagious after the first week, but instead is a "post-infectious" dry cough because of airway inflammation and mucous production.

Your child can return to school or daycare once the fever has disappeared and general symptoms are improving. This is roughly days 5 to 7 after the onset of symptoms.

 ## Home Care

The goals for treating bronchiolitis are to make your child comfortable, to lessen respiratory effort, and to observe carefully for deterioration. We ask you to read the entire "Home Care" section through first and select those recommendations that make the most sense for your child's situation.

1. Medication. Some children with bronchiolitis may respond to asthma medications, such as albuterol, levalbuterol, or similar drugs. This medicine is a bronchodilator; it helps open the airways by relaxing the smooth muscle spasms in the airway wall. If your child responds to this prescription medication, you may need to use the medicine for several days. It is best to call your health-care provider for a plan specific to the age of your child and the severity of the symptoms.

   If the wheezing recurs and is not an emergency, restart the medicine in the same dose and call your health-care provider the next day for further advice. If you have been so instructed, you may start treatment with a bronchodilator for the wheezing before you call. Then, assess your child's response to the treatment, and call the next day for further instructions.

   In addition, your child may be given ibuprofen or acetaminophen as directed for discomfort (for example, aching muscles, headache, etc.).

2. Hydration/feedings. Strongly encourage your child to drink adequate clear liquids. Milk and other dairy products should be avoided. Hydration

is essential, but if your child refuses all but formula or breast milk, try diluting the formula with water to reduce its concentration and thus its mucous-producing effect. You can also add water to pumped breast milk. Pedialyte®, Sleepy Time Tea®, Gatorade®, and other clear liquids are all fine. The better hydrated your child, the thinner your child's mucous, and the easier it is for your child to expel or mobilize mucous.

Coughing spasms are often caused by mucous secretions in the throat and airway. Warm liquids such as teas may loosen secretions and relax your child.

3. Humidification. Breathing warm, moist air helps loosen the mucous that interferes with breathing. Use a humidifier, especially in the bedroom and play area. You can use a cool or warm air humidifier or a steam vaporizer and have your child inhale the warm mist.

4. Nasal suction. If your child's nose is congested, he will have trouble breast-feeding or drinking from a bottle. The mucous membranes of the nose may be swollen, and thick mucous can accumulate to further block nasal airflow. Suction alone may not easily remove these secretions. Warm saltwater nose drops may loosen mucous. Place 2 or 3 drops of warm salt water in each nostril. Let the salt water settle for a minute or two, and then use a suction bulb syringe to pull out the mucous. You can repeat this procedure 3 or 4 times per day, until your child's nose becomes less congested. Too frequent suctioning, however, can worsen nasal congestion by causing a "rebound" of more swelling. The nasal drops often stimulate sneezing, which is another good way to expel nasal mucous.

5. Nasal spray. Nasal saline sprays are effective in infants and children of all ages. Suctioning of mucous after spraying may then be easier. The spray may also trigger a good, strong sneeze. Be gentle in spraying the solution up your child's nose.

6. Sleep. Sleep is essential for healing. It may be necessary to give a one-time dose of a cough suppressant (such as Delsym®) at bedtime only, to allow adequate sleep for restful healing. We strongly discourage the use of cough suppressants during the day. It is better for your child to cough up mucous and expel it from the respiratory tract than for the mucous to remain in the airways only to further thicken.

Attempt to raise the head of your child's bed to provide better mucous drainage. It may be difficult to maintain that head position, but it's worth a try.

TLC, especially at bedtime, is very important. Your child will relax, breathe easier, and sleep better if you can spend a little extra time cuddling him. You can often soothe anxiety and pain with your gentle touch.

7. Antihistamines/decongestants. We strongly discourage the use of these products for bronchiolitis. While there may a very short period of symptom relief with them, they can also thicken mucous, making it difficult to expel from the airway. We believe that thicker mucous can contribute directly to the development of secondary bacterial infections, such as bronchitis, ear infections, and sinusitis.

8. No smoking. Tobacco smoke aggravates wheezing and all respiratory symptoms and should be strictly forbidden in the house, especially when your child is ill. Smoke adheres to clothing, too, so clothes exposed to smoke should be removed from your child's presence, as well.

9. Antibiotics. Antibiotics are not useful in bronchiolitis unless there is a secondary bacterial complication.

Integrated Therapies

(Please refer to the section on "Administering Integrated Treatments" on page 19 for guidance on using any of the therapies that follow.)

AROMATHERAPY

- Aromatherapy with either eucalyptus radiata or ravensara aromatica, combined with mandarin may soothe the symptoms of bronchiolitis during an attack. You may make a preparation by adding 2 to 3 drops of each essential oil to 1 ounce of carrier oil and then massage into the soles of your child's feet. You may also administer them by steam inhalation or a bath. In general it is best to avoid other aromatherapies during the treatment of bronchiolitis.

HERBAL REMEDIES (For quick reference please refer to the "Herbal Remedies List" on page 31 and the inside cover.)

- Horehound may be very effective in reducing mucous production and improving a wet cough. It may help in the recuperative phase of bronchiolitis if there is a significant amount of mucous production. For dosing, follow the package labeling accurately.
- Valerian root is a mild herbal sedative that may offer some help in easing a child with a significant cough. Valerian root may be most useful at bedtime. For dosing, follow the package labeling accurately.

HOMEOPATHIC REMEDIES (For quick reference please refer to the "Homeopathic Remedies List" on page 32 and the inside cover.)

- A homeopathic remedy designed to resolve bronchial irritation and cough (manifesting as a deep chest cough), especially those associated with an asthma exacerbation, may be useful. The remedy can be taken 2 to 3 times daily during the acute illness and continued for up to 1 to 4 weeks after, as indicated by the persistence of the cough. (Respiratory 1)
- A homeopathic remedy designed to reduce bronchial spasm and wheezing, especially if associated with an asthma exacerbation, may be useful. The remedy can be taken 2 to 3 times daily during the acute illness and continued for up to 1 to 4 weeks after, as indicated by the persistence of the cough. (Respiratory 2)
- A homeopathic remedy designed to support the defense systems in viral infections may be useful. It can be taken 3 to 6 times daily when the virus is active (for example, fever, lethargy, etc.). (General Support 1)

BACH FLOWER REMEDIES

- Rescue Remedy™ may be of use if your child is uncomfortable from the illness, stress, or anxiety. You may use 2 drops every 10 minutes to every few hours to calm restlessness as needed.
- A lukewarm bath with 10 drops of Rescue Remedy™ added to the bathwater is often very effective at relieving agitation and stress in general.

NUTRITIONALS AND SUPPLEMENTS

- Vitamin A
- Vitamin C
- Vitamin E
- EFAs
- Zinc

DIETARY GUIDELINES

- Avoid dairy and citrus.
- Give small, frequent, nutritious snacks.
- Avoid sugary foods and fried foods.
- Warm, clear-based soups are particularly soothing.

INTEGRATIVE SUPPORTIVE CARE

- Please read the section on "Integrated Management of Respiratory Illness."

 ## When to Call Your Health-care Provider

Call immediately if any of the following occur:

- Shortness of breath or rapid breathing rate (over 60 breaths per minute in an infant or over 40 breaths per minute in children over the age of 2 years), especially in the absence of fever.
- Blueness of lips, mucous membranes, or fingernails.
- Long pauses between breaths (more than 5 to 10 seconds) in infants.
- Spasms that cause choking, passing out, or persistent vomiting.
- Blood in sputum or mucous.
- Vomiting blood.
- Wheezing that is worsening.
- Increasing lethargy with difficulty arousing your child.
- Signs of increasing dehydration. See "Dehydration" section.

Call within 24 hours if:

- Mild wheezing is not gone in 24 hours.
- Croupy, "barking seal" type cough with stridor (harsh breathing on inspiration) develops. See "Croup" section.
- Sustained increase in breathing rate for 4 hours (greater than 40 breaths per minute), especially when there is no fever causing the rapid breathing.
- Fever lasts more than 96 hours.
- Child less than 3 months old has worsening cough lasting over 72 hours.
- Chest pain in older children.
- Cough lasts over one week and is not getting better.
- Cough interferes with sleep or causes several days of missed school.
- The cough takes a dramatic turn for the worse.

BRONCHIOLITIS

 ## Other Relevant Sections

Asthma

Colds

Cough

Croup

Dehydration

Fever

Integrated Management of Respiratory Illnesses

 ## Prevention

Because the viruses (especially RSV) that cause bronchiolitis are highly contagious, exposure to other ill children and adults should be avoided when possible, especially during epidemic times of year. Very young infants are especially susceptible. Daycare centers, health club nurseries, and recreation centers are all breeding grounds and points of contact for the virus. Careful hand-washing is essential to prevent spread. Encourage your child to wash his hands frequently and keep fingers out of his mouth.

Description/Physiology

Bronchitis is an inflammation of the larger bronchial airways. It can be caused by a virus, bacteria, or an allergy. It often begins with typical cold symptoms, such as cough, runny nose, and low-grade fever. The cough usually becomes more productive, initially with clear mucous and then yellow and sometimes green sputum. Appetite and energy levels may decrease.

The cough is the main symptom of bronchitis. Coughing is the best way to expel mucous. While it is an irritating symptom, the cough remains an important protective mechanism for your child. While most coughs triggered by viruses, allergies, or environmental irritants will resolve on their own or respond well to simple treatments, the cough of bronchitis usually requires some form of treatment.

 ## Causes/Epidemiology

The vast majority of bronchitis from infectious causes is viral. Nevertheless, the general public believes most bronchitis is bacterial, and that is simply not the case in children. Bacterial bronchitis is relatively uncommon in children, although it is often over-diagnosed and thus over-treated. Too often, the principles of diagnosis and treatment for adults are applied to children. Bronchitis is a perfect example of this.

A bronchitis-like syndrome can also be caused by an allergy and can produce identical symptoms.

 ## Expected Course

Viral bronchitis is essentially a bad cold. The larger airways are inflamed, as are the mucous membranes of the nose and mouth. These cold symptoms, runny nose, etc., last approximately one week; then there will be a period of slow recovery. The cough may linger for 4 to 6 weeks after the onset of the illness. Please see the "Colds" section.

We suspect bacterial bronchitis in the child or adolescent who (1) has had at least a week of cough followed by an abrupt worsening of the cough, and (2) this worsening of the cough is accompanied by fever.

During examination with the stethoscope, we hear specific sounds in the lungs called "rhonchi," which are diagnostic of bronchitis. Once bacterial bronchitis is diagnosed, antibiotics can be prescribed—not for the primary viral illness, but to cure the secondary bacterial infection in the "bronchi" (larger airways).

Although you may suspect the diagnosis of bronchitis from your child's symptoms, your health-care provider must confirm the diagnosis. Several other illnesses have symptoms similar to bronchitis and are treated differently.

It is important to remember that not all symptoms of bacterial bronchitis will resolve while your child is on antibiotics. This is because the antibiotic is responsible for killing the invading bacteria but is not responsible for healing the irritated tissue. As with viral bronchitis, the initial symptoms may persist for 1 to 2 weeks. In many children, there appears to be a "post-infection phase" while the body is repairing irritated tissue, during which time the cough may linger, persisting in a milder form for one to several weeks more.

In true bacterial bronchitis, we strongly recommend a re-check of the lungs within a week after antibiotics have been stopped, to confirm that the lungs are clear.

Bronchitis rarely develops into a more serious illness such as pneumonia, but it is important to watch your child for abrupt changes of symptoms, including a worsening of cough, higher fever, more-labored breathing, or wheezing. Because pneumonia and asthma may also present with these symptoms, all children with this worsening respiratory pattern should be evaluated medically.

Contagiousness/Immunity

Bacterial bronchitis is not typically contagious. It is difficult to transmit the bacteria from one person to another, although it is possible in certain instances. However, the virus that causes a viral bronchitis can be spread to another child. Chances are, however, the newly infected child will not develop anything more than a cold from the same virus.

Some children seem to be particularly prone to developing bronchitis. The reasons are not always clear, but may pertain to differences in individual anatomy and immune response: increased exposure rates in some children to viral illnesses (daycare) or an allergic/irritant component due, for example, to cigarette smoke exposure. Some of these children with a history of "recurrent bronchitis" may later be diagnosed as having asthma. Your health-care provider can help assess your child's individual history and, if necessary, develop an appropriate treatment plan.

Home Care

The goals for treatment are to provide comfort for your child, relieve the cough, prevent spread of the disease, and provide a cure if the bronchitis is bacterial. Please read through the entire "Home Care" section first to select those recommendations that make the most sense for your child's situation.

- Eliminate dairy intake for 5 days (all dairy—not just milk). Increase clear fluids as much as possible. Hydration is always a key to faster recovery. Drink a lot of clear liquids!
- Use a vaporizer or humidifier (cool or steam) continuously at night.
- Use a mild cough suppressant if the cough is disrupting sleep. See "OTC Medication Recommendations and Dosages" section.
- An antibiotic may be prescribed as part of the home regimen after the diagnosis has been made by your health-care provider.
- If there is a wheezing component, a bronchodilator such as albuterol may be of some benefit. This treatment is best directed by your health-care provider.
- Adequate rest and sleep are essential for full recovery. Some limited activity does allow better mobilization of mucous, however.

 Integrated Therapies

(Please refer to the section on "Administering Integrated Treatments" on page 19 for guidance on using any of the therapies that follow.)

AROMATHERAPY

- Add 2 drops of the essential oil of eucalyptus radiata to 1 to 2 teaspoons of olive oil and rub on your child's chest to soothe a cough or congestion.
- An aromatherapy bath or massage with the essential oils of eucalyptus radiata and/or lavender can soothe and relax your child's anxiety and restlessness as well as his congestion and difficult breathing. Add 2 to 5 drops of oil to a warm bath and allow your child to soak for a comfortable period of time.

HERBAL REMEDIES (For quick reference please refer to the "Herbal Remedies List" on page 31 and the inside cover.)

- Cherry bark may be very effective in reducing the dry irritative cough that frequently follows a bronchial infection. For dosing, follow the package labeling accurately.

- Horehound may be very effective in reducing mucous production and improving a wet cough. It may help in the recuperative phase of bronchitis, if there is a significant amount of mucous production. For dosing, follow the package labeling accurately.
- Valerian root is a mild herbal sedative that may offer some help in easing a child with a significant cough. Valerian root may be most useful at bedtime. For dosing, follow the package labeling accurately.

HOMEOPATHIC REMEDIES (For quick reference please refer to the "Homeopathic Remedies List" on page 32 and the inside cover.)

- A homeopathic remedy designed to resolve bronchial irritation and coughs (manifesting as a deep chest cough), especially those associated with an asthma exacerbation, may be useful. The remedy can be taken 2 to 3 times daily during the acute illness and continued for up to 1 to 4 weeks after, as indicated by the persistence of the cough. (Respiratory 1)
- A homeopathic remedy designed to support the defense systems in viral infections may be useful. It can be taken 3 to 6 times daily when the virus is active (for example, fever, lethargy, etc.). (General Support 1)
- A homeopathic remedy designed to decrease inflammation and fever from infections may help prevent deterioration and improve the recovery time. It can be taken 3 to 6 times daily when the virus is active (for example, fever, lethargy, etc.). (General Support 2)

BACH FLOWER REMEDIES

- Rescue Remedy™ may be of use if your child has anxiety with episodes of coughing. You may use 2 drops every 10 minutes to every few hours to calm restlessness as needed.

NUTRITIONALS AND SUPPLEMENTS

- Vitamin A
- Vitamin C
- EFAs
- Zinc

DIETARY GUIDELINES

- Avoid mucous-forming foods, especially all dairy products and citrus fruits and their juices.

- Give small, frequent, nutritious snacks.
- Avoid sugary foods and fried foods.
- Warm soups are particularly soothing.

INTEGRATIVE SUPPORTIVE CARE

- Please read the section "Integrated Management of Respiratory Illnesses."

 ## When to Call Your Health-care Provider

Call immediately if any of the following occur:

- Shortness of breath or rapid breathing rate (over 60 breaths per minute in an infant or over 40 breaths per minute in children over the age of 2 years), especially in the absence of fever.
- Blueness of lips, mucous membranes, or fingernails.
- Spasms that cause choking, passing out, and/or persistent vomiting.
- Blood in sputum or mucous.
- Vomiting blood.
- Sudden onset of violent coughing in a child who might have aspirated (choked into the airway) a small object, such as food or a toy.
- Wheezing that is worsening.
- Intense chest pain with coughing.
- High fevers of more than 104 degrees associated with cough and respiratory distress.
- Progressive lethargy to the point of being difficult to arouse easily.
- Signs of dehydration have developed.

Call within 24 hours if:

- Mild wheezing persists for more than 24 hours.
- Croupy, "barking seal" type cough develops with any difficulty in breathing, especially stridor (harsh inspiratory breathing). See "Croup" section.
- There is a sustained increase in respiratory rate for 12 hours.
- Fever lasts more than 72 hours.
- Child is less than 3 months old with a cough lasting over 72 hours.

- Chest pain occurs in older children.
- Cough lasts more than 2 weeks without gradual improvement.
- Cough interferes with sleep without relief from above measures.
- Illness causes several days of missed school.

 ## Other Relevant Sections

Asthma

Bronchiolitis

Colds

Cough

Croup

Dehydration

Fever

Integrated Management of Respiratory Illnesses

 ## Prevention

True bacterial bronchitis (requiring antibiotics) is uncommon; however, other causative triggers are not. So, if your child is susceptible to bronchitis, pay particular attention to those obvious triggers which, in the past, have led to this secondary bronchitis diagnosis: allergy triggers, cigarette smoke, and viral infections. If your child does develop a cold or allergy symptoms, start treatment early, as recommended in this handbook, to help lessen the severity and duration of these symptoms. Early intervention can significantly reduce the progression of symptoms and possible bronchitis.

Description/Physiology

Chickenpox is a familiar, viral childhood illness caused by the varicella-zoster virus. In most children, chickenpox, while uncomfortable, is relatively benign. Today, with the advent of the chickenpox vaccine, we are seeing far fewer cases of the disease and its complications (skin infections and scarring).

The virus can be transmitted through the air and by infected secretions. It enters the respiratory tract through the mouth or nose and invades the mucous membranes. The virus rapidly multiplies and is spread by the bloodstream throughout the body. It has a predilection for these mucous membranes and the skin. In these areas it creates pockets of inflammation, mucous, and the characteristic pox lesion.

 ## Expected Course

Chickenpox is characterized by 2 to 3 days of early symptoms: fever, irritability, headache, loss of appetite, and cold-like symptoms (cough, runny nose, and red eyes). This "preview" is followed by the appearance of the distinctive chickenpox rash, and these early symptoms may continue along with the appearance of the pox.

The typical pox begins as a spot about the size of a medium-sized mosquito bite, usually on the trunk. Within 12 to 48 hours, these spots progress through several stages—from a blister-topped "mosquito bite" to a pus-filled pimple to a crust-topped sore. The pox typically break out in waves, with groups of new pox developing every 12 to 24 hours. They are generally scattered evenly over the entire body. They may break out for 3 to 10 days, and cases may vary from very mild (a few pox) to very severe (hundreds of lesions). These pox become blisters and eventually scab over. The scabs may remain on the skin up to 2 weeks, fall off, and reveal pinkish, healing skin underneath.

Pox may also occur in the genitals, eyes, ears, mouth, and throat. Chickenpox in these areas may require special care, and they can be particularly uncomfortable. Pox anywhere may itch intensely and may be painful. Many children develop enlargement of their lymph nodes, especially in the head and neck during the infection.

Chickenpox may leave permanent scars, but this occurs only in a small percentage of children. There is no evidence that pox are more likely to scar if your child repeatedly picks off the scabs. However, children are encouraged not to scratch these lesions (although this may be extremely difficult to enforce), because scratching may increase the risk of secondary infection. The scarring is more a function of the depth of the initial pox erosion and less from the actual scratching. The average chickenpox leaves a temporary mark on the skin, which usually fades in 6 to 12 months.

Complications of chickenpox are very rare but can be quite severe. Children may develop infected pox, and this can cause generalized skin infections, such as cellulitis or impetigo. Pox in the mouth can reduce fluid intake, so watch for dehydration. See "Dehydration" section. There are much rarer complications of chickenpox, such as deep-tissue bacterial infections, Reye's Syndrome (associated with taking aspirin), pneumonia, and encephalitis.

 ## Contagiousness/Immunity

Chickenpox is highly contagious, transmitted through direct contact with the active pox, through airborne contact, and through exchanges of oral and nasal secretions. Your infected child is contagious for 2 to 3 days before the rash breaks out and until all the pox have crusted over (usually 5 to 10 days). The incubation period can be as short as 7 days from the first day of exposure to as long as 21 days from the last day of exposure. The incubation period is usually 14 to 21 days.

Both mild and severe cases provide equal immunity for life. Very, very rarely, a child may develop a second, mild case of chickenpox. When this does happen, we are suspicious that the initial diagnosis of chickenpox may not have been accurate, or the child may have been too young (less than 12 months of age) to form full immunity.

As you know, there is a vaccine against chickenpox called Varivax®. With the majority of children now receiving this vaccine, there has been a dramatic decline in the number of primary cases of chickenpox. The vaccine itself generally prevents the disease altogether; however, in a small number of instances, an exposed child who has been immunized may develop a mild form of chickenpox. This vaccine is both safe and highly effective.

Parents themselves who have not had chickenpox are strongly encouraged to consult their own physician for this vaccine. The older child and adult are more likely to have a serious infection and secondary complications as noted above.

It is possible for an unvaccinated child to contract chickenpox from a patient with shingles (herpes zoster), but only if they are in direct contact with the shingles lesions, because unlike chickenpox, shingles is not contagious through the air. A child cannot contract shingles from a patient with shingles, because shingles is a "reactivation" of one's own earlier chickenpox infection.

Home Care

Most of the unpleasant symptoms of chickenpox can be soothed and largely relieved. However, there is often a degree of misery that will not respond to any medical treatment and will require a focused amount of your tender loving care. Our goals for treatment are relief of discomfort, prevention of spread of the disease, and good hydration. Please read through the entire "Home Care" section first to determine which of our recommendations make the most sense for your child's situation.

1. Fever and aches. You may treat with acetaminophen or ibuprofen. Please see the "Fever" section and "OTC Drug Recommendations and Dosages" section.

   NOTE: DO NOT USE ANY ASPIRIN-CONTAINING PRODUCTS.

2. Itching control:

   A. A cool bath with baking soda or colloidal oatmeal (Aveeno®) are extremely helpful, though this provides only short-lasting relief. To dry your child, pat, don't rub.

   B. Calamine cream may be applied directly to the pox as often as necessary to control itching.

   C. Benadryl® (syrup or tablets) may be taken orally. Please see the "OTC Medication Recommendations and Dosages" section. Benadryl sprays are also available. Be careful not to use oral Benadryl® and any topical products containing Benadryl® at the same time.

   D. Soak a flannel-type pajama in water and wring it out well. Have your child put on these pajamas and then put on a dry pair over them. The slow evaporation will cool the skin and thus relieve itching.

3. Infection prevention. Prevent pox from becoming infected by keeping your child's fingernails short and clean. Wearing gloves or socks on hands may help prevent digging. Discourage scratching, especially the face. Washing hands with an antibacterial soap (Dial®, Safeguard®) may help.

4. Mouth sores. For mouth sores, encourage cold fluids and offer a soft, bland diet. Avoid salty foods and citrus fruits. Popsicles, fruit juices, and herbal teas are very soothing. If the mouth ulcers worsen, have your child rinse his mouth or gargle with one tablespoon of an antacid solution (for example, Maalox® or Mylanta®) after meals and snacks. Painful oral pox

may reduce drinking, and dehydration may result. See "Dehydration" section. Usually you can stay ahead of dehydration by constant offers and reminders of fluids.

5. Vaginal ulcers. Vaginal ulcers may be very painful and interfere with urination. Calamine lotion applied to the labia is fine, or you may try a thin layer of Vaseline®. These two preparations can be applied several times per day.

6. Medication changes. If your child takes steroid medications (Pediapred®, Prelone®, Prednisone®, Decadron®) and has been exposed to chickenpox, call your health-care provider to discuss medication changes and how to proceed.

7. Sunscreen. Please be sure to put plenty of sunscreen on your child after all chickenpox infections.

 Integrated Therapies

(Please refer to the section on "Administering Integrated Treatments" on page 19 for guidance on using any of the therapies that follow.)

AROMATHERAPY

• An aromatherapy bath or massage with the essential oils of eucalyptus radiata and/or lavender can soothe and relax your child's anxiety and restlessness. Add 2 to 5 drops of oil to a warm bath and allow your child to soak for a comfortable period of time.

HERBAL REMEDIES (For quick reference please refer to the "Herbal Remedies List" on page 31 and the inside cover.)

• Echinacea/astragalus can be used to support the immune system in helping to resolve a viral infection. For dosing, follow the package labeling accurately.

• Valerian root is a mild herbal sedative that may offer some help in easing a child with a significant restlessness. Valerian root may be most useful at bedtime and occasionally for a nap. For dosing, follow the package labeling accurately.

• Aloe vera or calendula applied topically can reduce itching and soothe irritated skin. They are available in gel, lotion, or cream. For dosing, follow the package labeling accurately.

• Sponge-bathing your child with infusion strength peppermint tea can be very soothing to his skin.

HOMEOPATHIC REMEDIES (For quick reference please refer to the "Homeopathic Remedies List" on page 32 and the inside cover.)

• A homeopathic remedy designed to support the defense systems in viral infections may be useful. It can be taken 3 to 6 times daily when the virus is active (for example, fever, lethargy, etc.). (General Support 1)

• A homeopathic cream designed to soothe inflamed or irritated skin may be useful. It may also promote skin healing and minimize scarring. It may be gently rubbed directly onto the pox 2 to 3 times a day. (Skin 1)

• A homeopathic remedy designed to relieve some of the discomforts associated with infections (for example, fever, body aches, chills, and fatigue) may be useful. It can be taken 3 to 6 times daily when the virus is active (for example, fever, lethargy, etc.). (General Support 3)

BACH FLOWER REMEDIES

• Rescue Remedy™ may be of use if your child is uncomfortable from the illness, stress, or anxiety. You may use 2 drops every 10 minutes to every few hours to calm restlessness as needed.

• Ten drops of Rescue Remedy™ added to a lukewarm bath is often very effective at relieving many of the symptoms of the chickenpox.

NUTRITIONALS AND SUPPLEMENTS

• Vitamin E can be used topically to speed skin healing and minimize scarring. Take a vitamin E gel cap and poke a hole in it and then squeeze some onto your finger and rub it directly onto the pox. This may be done once or twice daily until the area is healed.

When to Call Your Health-care Provider

Call immediately if:

- Any pox appears to be infected. You will see an enlarging red ring (one inch or larger) around the pox. There may be pus drainage from this infected pox or extreme tenderness.
- The pox appear anywhere on the globe of the eye itself. Pox on the eyelid itself are not a problem, however. The eyes are often red from the general illness, but an actual pox on the eyeball should prompt an immediate call. The presence of a pox on the eye itself may not be easily determined except by an exam or with an ophthalmologist's evaluation.
- Your child develops persistent vomiting, is difficult to arouse, or is confused. This caution is especially true 7 to 14 days after the illness has resolved.
- Your child develops symptoms of dehydration: a very dry mouth, no urine in 12 hours, no tears with crying, etc.
- Your child is less than 4 months of age.
- Your child develops a stiff neck, has trouble walking, or is disoriented.
- A mother develops chickenpox within two weeks of delivering a newborn, as the infant may require special medications to prevent a serious case of chickenpox.

Call within 24 hours if:

- Any of the milder symptoms need more specific relief than afforded by the above recommendations.
- Your child develops a lymph node (gland) that is large, red, or tender.
- You would like help in confirming the diagnosis.

 ## Other Relevant Sections

Colds

Conjunctivitis (Pinkeye with Pus)

Cough

Dehydration

Fever

Impetigo

 ## Prevention

Prevention is best accomplished through the Varicella Vaccine or Varivax®. In addition, avoid children with diagnosed chickenpox. Chickenpox is highly contagious by direct contact as well as airborne. Always use good hand-washing after you have handled your child in any way. The virus can survive on inanimate objects, such as toys, for several hours. You should wash your hands after handling objects touched by your child.

It is possible to transmit the virus on your unwashed hands for a period of several hours after you have contaminated your hands. In this way, you do not have to have the infection yourself to pass it along.

If your child needs to be seen by your health-care provider or the emergency room, be sure to advise the staff in advance that you suspect chickenpox so that your child can be isolated in a special room. This will prevent exposure of other children and parents in the waiting room and exam areas.

Description/Physiology

The cold is the most common illness in childhood. On average, your child may suffer up to 6 to 8 minor upper respiratory infections (colds) per year. Older children may have 3 to 5 colds per year.

The most typical symptoms of a cold are runny nose, congestion, cough, sore throat, lethargy, ear congestion, sneezing, swollen lymph glands (especially in the neck), and fever-associated aches. In infants and young children, their discomfort is further intensified by their inability to handle mucous production in the same ways that adults do—by blowing the nose or coughing up mucous.

Also, a child's smaller nasal passages are more easily blocked by mucous membrane swelling and mucous production. To complicate matters further, dry climates are an irritant to the membranes of the airways, since dryness will slow the healing process.

Causes/Epidemiology

Colds are caused by viruses. There is no cure for the common cold. Antibiotics are of absolutely no use in viral colds. Eventually, your child's own immune system will eliminate the infecting virus.

In a given winter season, there may be several viruses active in the community at any one time. It is common for a child to acquire a second viral infection right on the heels of a first, making the entire period of illness stretch up to 15 to 20 days. It may appear as if this is one, very long-lasting cold when, in fact, it is probably two separate infections with two different viruses infecting your child back-to-back.

Once in a while, the cause of a runny nose (especially one-sided, thick, mucous discharge) can be a foreign body stuck up the nose. In addition, overuse of nasal sprays (other than homeopathic) can also produce a pattern of recurrent nasal discharge and cold-like symptoms.

Expected Course

The average duration of acute cold symptoms is 5 to 10 days. A fever is often present, lasting on average 3 to 4 days. The fever can range from 100 to 104 degrees. The cough is a prominent symptom. The duration of a cough associated with a cold is usually one week, but the cough may persist up to one month.

The mucous of a runny nose from a cold is initially clear to white. Over a few days, however, it may develop into a yellow and even a green mucous. Yellow and green mucous are still signs of a viral illness unless these colors persist for more than 2 weeks. The yellow and green discharge is part of the healing phase of most viruses, and just a few days of green or yellow discharge does not mean that your child now has a bacterial infection, for example, a sinus infection. This is a common misconception. This "over-diagnosis" of a bacterial infection often leads to over-treatment with antibiotics.

There can be several complications of the common cold. Pneumonia and bronchitis from viruses or bacteria are possible, though not likely. There can be secondary infections such as ear infections, bacterial conjunctivitis, sinusitis, and impetigo.

 ## Contagiousness/Immunity

Colds are transmitted only by direct contact with someone else who has a cold. In addition, a child who has been physically stressed by cold air, sleep deprivation, poor diet, cigarette smoke, and emotional stress may be more susceptible to the invading virus. Look for stress triggers (see "Stress" section) in your child's life that might disrupt your child's healthy life balance. You will learn your own child's sensitivity to environmental stresses, and you should provide appropriate protection and prevention techniques.

Cold viruses are quite contagious. Your child is contagious throughout all symptoms, but especially during the presence of fever. If all that remains of a cold is a cough, contagiousness is minimal. The average period of contagiousness is 5 to 7 days. A child may be contagious up to 2 days before the first symptoms develop.

 ## Home Care

The primary goals for treatment of colds are to relieve discomfort, enhance sleep, reduce spread of the infection to others, and speed recovery.

The general stresses that may trigger a cold (changes in activity, nutrition, and sleep) are very important and often overlooked. Think carefully about your child's entire environment, and see if the elimination of certain stresses might improve your child's overall health.

Please read through the entire "Home Care" section first to select those recommendations that make the most sense for your child's situation.

1. Activity. A child usually imposes his own appropriate restrictions on activity during the first several days of a cold; however, once he is beginning to feel better, your child needs close supervision to manage his activity level. Severe activity restrictions are not required; however, it is appropriate to protect your child from overexertion (for example, indoor versus outdoor play). Children are quick to return to their normal activity, often prematurely, and so healing energy is diverted to play energy.

2. Sleep. Sleep, like activity, tends to take care of itself during the first several days of a cold. Once your child is beginning to feel better, however, it is beneficial to encourage 30 to 60 minutes of extra sleep in a 24-hour period. Normal sleep patterns may be restored in 1 to 2 weeks. If coughing, fever, etc., are disturbing your child's sleep, please see "Fever" and "Cough" sections.

3. Diet. Nutritional requirements vary during a cold. Throughout the cold and its resolution process, it is essential that good fluid intake be maintained. Good fluid intake will help keep mucous thinner.

   In older children (over 12 months), milk and all other dairy products should be avoided for approximately 5 days. Milk products stimulate the increased production of mucous. Formula-fed infants under 12 months may benefit from 1 or 2 days of diluted formula. See "Dehydration" section. Breast-fed infants and babies should continue their regular routine.

   Many children will have almost no appetite for solid foods during the first several days of a cold. This is normal and represents no danger to them. Once your child begins to feel better, his appetite will improve. Since digestion is made more difficult by the cold, the diet should be kept light. Foods with a high fat content, such as peanut butter, fried foods, dairy products, and meats, should be kept to a minimum. Limit sugary foods, as well.

4. Environment. Your child should be kept warm while he is recovering from a cold. When your child becomes cold, he uses much energy to maintain body temperature. This energy could be devoted to healing instead of temperature regulation.

5. Nasal congestion. Congestion and cough are generally the last cold symptoms to disappear. Initially, blowing the nose and wiping the nostrils free of mucous, and then applying Vaseline®, Bag Balm®, Ayr Gel or Calendula cream (available at most health food stores) to inflamed nasal tissue for protection are the main lines of support. You may also:

   A. Increase oral fluid intake. Herbal teas such as mint and chamomile may help.

B. Use a bulb syringe. In small children, clear nostrils with a bulb syringe and use saline nose drops made of $1/2$ teaspoon of salt and 1 cup of water or commercially available saline drops (for example, Ocean®). Put 2 drops in each nostril and suction away mucous. Repeat as needed 3 to 4 times per day. Nasal suctioning too frequently can cause a "rebound" of worsening congestion.

If nasal congestion is significantly interfering with eating or sleeping and saline nose drops are not sufficient, you may consider using OTC phenylephrine nose drops in a strength of $1/8$% or $1/4$%. You may administer 1 to 2 drops in each nostril as needed to support eating and sleeping, for a maximum of 3 doses per day for a maximum of 7 days. (Use for longer periods can result in nasal membrane dependency.)

C. Use humidifiers. Either cool-mist or warm-mist humidifiers/vaporizers are fine. We find both equally effective. Keep humidifiers/vaporizers clean according to the manufacturer's instructions. (NOTE: If warm mist or steam vaporizers are used, monitor your child closely to prevent accidental skin burns.)

D. Nasal washes. For older children, nasal washes with saline (as in B above) can loosen thickened secretions. Put 3 to 4 drops of a nasal wash into each nostril and wait for a minute or two before blowing.

6. Use of decongestants/antihistamines. We are generally opposed to their use for colds. Both preparations tend to thicken the mucous. This makes it flow less freely and thus the mucous is more susceptible to bacterial overgrowth. This then increases the risk of secondary infections, such as sinus and ear infections. We prefer the natural approach first, as detailed above. Oftentimes, oral decongestants make children irritable, restless, and even agitated. The benefits are not worth the side effects.

7. Coughs. Coughs are designed to clear mucous from the airway and thus help protect your child from developing an infection in the lower airways (pneumonia, bronchitis). We recommend cough suppressants be reserved for coughs which significantly disturb sleeping and eating. When cough suppressants are required, we recommend a dextromethorphan preparation such as Delsym®. Please see the "OTC Medication Recommendations and Dosages" section. Also, chest vaporubs may provide some relief.

8. Aches and pains. The aches and pains caused by colds and fevers are uncomfortable but usually short-lived. Extra rest and cuddling will often bring relief. Acetaminophen or ibuprofen will also help. See the "OTC Medication Recommendations and Dosages" section.

9. Sore throat. A sore throat is often part of the common cold. When present, it is often the main focus of your child's attention. Humidification, fluids, popsicles, throat lozenges, and throat sprays will all provide some relief. Preparations such as Throat Coat Tea® and Ricola® lozenges are helpful. See "Throat" section.

10. Red eyes. Cool compresses are best. See "Conjunctivitis" section.

11. Fever discomfort. See "Fever" section.
    Note: Please avoid the use of aspirin or aspirin-containing products.

 Integrated Therapies

(Please refer to the section on "Administering Integrated Treatments" on page 19 for guidance on using any of the therapies that follow.)

AROMATHERAPY

• An aromatherapy bath or massage with the essential oils of eucalyptus radiata and/or lavender can soothe and relax your child's anxiety and restlessness as well as his congestion and difficult breathing. Add 2 to 5 drops of oil to a warm bath and allow your child to soak for a comfortable period of time.

• Add 2 drops each of the essential oils of eucalyptus radiata and lavender to 1 to 2 teaspoons of olive oil and rub on your child's chest to soothe a cough or congestion.

HERBAL REMEDIES (For quick reference please refer to the "Herbal Remedies List" on page 31 and the inside cover.)

• Horehound may be very effective in reducing mucous production and improving congestion and a wet cough. It may help in the recuperative phase of a cold if there is a significant amount of mucous production. For dosing, follow the package labeling accurately.

• Valerian root is a mild herbal sedative that may offer some help in easing a child with a significant cold. Valerian root may be most useful at bedtime. For dosing, follow the package labeling accurately.

• Echinacea/astragalus can be used to support the immune system in helping to resolve a viral infection. For dosing, follow the package labeling accurately.

• Beverage strength herbal teas may offer some soothing relief of cold symptoms (especially a sore throat) and also provides a good source of fluids. Herb teas made from chamomile or mint as well as a variety of blended herbal teas (refer to "Herbal Therapies" section) can be brewed according to package directions, sweetened to taste, and offered frequently through the day.

HOMEOPATHIC REMEDIES (For quick reference please refer to the "Homeopathic Remedies List" on page 32 and the inside cover.)

- A homeopathic remedy designed to minimize nasal congestion and mucous, especially when associated with respiratory infections, may be useful. It can be taken 2 to 3 times daily while there is nasal congestion. (Respiratory 3)
- A homeopathic remedy designed to reduce the symptoms of a common cold may be useful to provide some relief from the cold symptoms. It can be taken 2 to 3 times daily during the illness. (Respiratory 4)
- A homeopathic remedy designed to support the defense system in viral infections may be useful. It can be taken 3 to 6 times daily when the virus is active (for example, fever, lethargy, etc.). (General Support 1)
- A homeopathic remedy designed to decrease inflammation and fever from infections may help prevent deterioration and improve recovery time. It can be taken 3 to 6 times daily when the virus is active (for example, fever, lethargy, etc.). (General Support 2)

BACH FLOWER REMEDIES

- Rescue Remedy™ may be of use if your child is uncomfortable from the illness, stress, or anxiety. You may use 2 drops every 10 minutes to every few hours to calm restlessness as needed.
- A lukewarm bath with 10 drops of Rescue Remedy™ added to the bathwater is often very effective at relieving agitation and stress in general.

NUTRITIONALS AND SUPPLEMENTS

- Vitamin A
- Vitamin C
- Zinc

DIETARY GUIDELINES

- It is best to avoid all dairy products and citrus fruits because they may increase or thicken respiratory mucous.
- Warm foods such as soups, warm cooked grains (such as oatmeal), and teas should be given.
- Cold foods, foods high in sugar, and fried foods should be avoided.

INTEGRATIVE SUPPORTIVE CARE

- Please read the section "Integrated Management of Respiratory Illnesses."

 ## When to Call Your Health-care Provider

Call immediately if any of the following occur:

- Shortness of breath or rapid breathing rate (over 60 breaths per minute in an infant or over 40 breaths per minute in children over the age of 2 years), especially in the absence of fever.
- Significant chest pain in an older child.
- Fever of greater than 100.4 degrees rectal or 99.4 degrees under the arm is present in a child less than 2 months of age.
- Progressive lethargy in a child who is difficult to arouse.
- Progressive signs of dehydration because of decreased fluid intake or abnormal losses with vomiting or diarrhea. See "Dehydration" section.
- Fever that exceeds 105 degrees when taken with a rectal or oral thermometer (see "Fever" section).

Call within 24 hours if:

- Fever lasts more than 4 days.
- There is no improvement of symptoms after 7 full days.
- The skin in and around the nose becomes raw or cracked and develops gold crusting.
- Discharge from the nose becomes green and remains green for more than 14 days; 1 to 10 days of intermittent green nasal discharge is common.
- Fever returns in the middle of the cold.
- An earache develops.
- Heavy eye draining occurs, requiring removal of mucous every hour or two.

 ## Other Relevant Sections

Asthma

Bronchiolitis
Bronchitis
Conjunctivitis
Cough
Croup
Dehydration
Earache/Ear Infection
Fever
Sinus Infection
Sore Throat
Integrated Management of Respiratory Illnesses

 Prevention

The single most important prevention technique is careful hand-washing by all caretakers. The virus is easily transmitted through the oral and nasal secretions of an infected child or adult to another child through direct hand contact. The virus can live on the hand's surface for several hours. During respiratory season, caregivers should wash their hands frequently and especially after direct contact with a sick child (for example, wiping a nose, picking up used tissues, etc.).

Teach your children at an early age to wash their hands frequently when they are ill. They should be encouraged to keep their hands out of their mouth and away from their nose and eyes as much as possible. The virus is also transmitted through the air, so teach your children to cover their mouth and nose when sneezing and coughing and then to wash their hands after doing so. Hint: You may want to teach your child to cough into his arm/sleeve to minimize the airborne and contact spread of germs.

The virus can live on inanimate surfaces (toys, books) for a number of hours. Careful daily washing of play toys and washable books is important to control viral spread.

Avoid contact with children and adults who are known to be ill. This is especially important in children who are prone to other complications such as asthma, croup, and pneumonia and also for those with more serious chronic illnesses such as diabetes. Daycare centers, health club nurseries, and preschools are prime sites for viral spread. Your respectful decision to keep your own ill child home will reduce viral spread at these centers.

COLIC AND THE FUSSY BABY

 ## Description/Physiology

Many babies develop symptoms of colic in the early months of life. Colic is described as extreme irritability which is difficult to control by normal means (for example, cuddling, feeding, etc.). The crying may be very intense or for long periods (more than three hours a day) or both. Naturally, most babies have fussy periods, but colic is characterized by more extreme crying, especially in the late afternoon and evening. Roughly 25 percent of infants have some form of colic.

Babies can swallow a good deal of air with feedings and with crying, and this swallowed air may further add to your baby's gas problems or indigestion. Oftentimes you will see your baby writhe in pain, with an arched back, a red face, and flailing arms. The onset of crying may be abrupt and without warning and with no obvious trigger. These babies often act fine in between bouts of crying, and they are not usually sick in any other way.

You may become very frustrated, anxious, depressed, sleep-deprived, and exhausted. In fact, this can be one of the most trying times for new parents.

 ## Causes/Epidemiology

There are two types of colicky babies:

1. Those colicky babies whose crying seems to be closely associated with feedings, regardless of the time of day. These babies tend to fuss after most feedings, have problems with gas, have gurgling bowel sounds, and frequently quiet down after a brief stretch of sleep. They may remain quiet until the next feeding. It is presumed that these babies develop colic because of difficulty with digestion due to an immature digestive tract and/or food intolerance, whether formula or breast milk.

   This type of colic may also be triggered by "gastroesophageal reflux" disease, or GERD. This is the equivalent of "heartburn" in adults. The acid produced in the stomach by normal digestion moves backwards up the esophagus and causes irritation and pain in the esophagus. Many of these infants have significant spitting up, although some have no visible spitting up at all. This stomach acid weakens the valve (sphincter) that guards the esophagus from the stomach, further lessening its tightening function.

2. Those colicky babies who tend to cry at specific, isolated times of the day, unrelated to any obvious environmental activity. They are usually fussy in the evenings or nights, but they don't usually have significant

symptoms of indigestion such as gas or gurgling. It is felt that these babies are suffering from "environmental overstimulation" and they usually respond best to quiet, soothing activities (see below).

These two types of colic are not distinct and separate. Therefore, the measures we suggest to improve their fussing often overlap, as well.

Expected Course

Colic usually begins between the second and fourth weeks of life, peaks at 6 to 10 weeks, and will usually last several months. You will see many, many suggestions listed below to help you until your child naturally outgrows this tendency. It is rare for a child to be colicky after six months; however, certain babies remain fussy for several additional months, depending on the cause.

Home Care

Ask for help—friends, neighbors, and your health-care providers! You must also pay attention to your own personal needs for rest, exercise, and nutrition.

Please observe your baby carefully for timing and feeding clues that might help your health-care provider craft an approach specific to the needs of your child. Create an awake/sleep/feeding/crying/elimination log to accurately record your baby's daily behaviors. In this way, you can identify trends, triggers, and patterns that can help your health-care provider anticipate colic episodes.

We encourage you to try all of the suggestions listed below. Very importantly, we also encourage you to call your health-care provider with the details of your child's colic and what you have already tried so that they can help you. All babies outgrow colic, but these can be difficult months, especially if you feel isolated in coping with your fussy baby. Having a colicky baby can be very frustrating. Not only is it exhausting, it is also very complicated emotionally. As parents we feel we should be able to soothe our infants when they are unhappy. The exhaustion we have from coping with our infant's colic is compounded by the feeling that we are failures as parents. This can lead to resentment of the infant, which further compounds our feelings with a sense of guilt. Furthermore, we are struggling with these complicated emotions while we are exhausted. Thus, it would be ideal to develop and use a group of family, friends, and professional caregivers to provide you a much-needed break.

Please read the entire "Home Care" section first to select those recommendations that make the most sense for your child's current situation.

1. For those babies whose colic appears primarily digestive (See Type 1 above), you may try the following:

   A. It is very important to differentiate between hunger discomfort and colic pain. If you're convinced the discomfort is due to hunger, you should attend to the hunger signal as quickly as possible. If, however, you believe that the distress is coming from "colicky pain," it is better to comfort your infant without feeding him, as feeding could increase the colic in the long run. It is better to stretch out the feedings to minimize the cramps that can arise from feeding. Feedings should be given in a comfortable, quiet, soothing environment.

   B. Place warm water bottles on the "tummy" after each feeding. Protect direct skin contact with a thin towel or diaper.

   C. Plan to spend extra time after the feeding cuddling and nurturing your baby.

   D. Give your baby one to two ounces of peppermint, spearmint, or Sleepy Time® tea (Celestial Seasonings), brewed lightly, served warm. You may offer this 2 to 3 times per day during peak crying episodes. (NOTE: Do not give peppermint extract, as it can be toxic to infants.)

   E. Dietary changes:
      (1) When breast-feeding, your baby may be sensitive to something in your diet, so try restricting your intake of common offenders like chocolate, caffeine, dairy products, spicy foods, and gassy vegetables (beans, onions, cabbage, peppers or broccoli).
         You might try eliminating some or all of these foods and carefully re-introduce each one back into your diet while observing your infant's reactions. Introduce one new food at a time every 2 to 3 days.
      (2) For formula-fed babies, the formula itself may be the problem. Please call your health-care provider for recommendations about a formula change. Also, check the hole in the nipple. Large and small holes both may contribute to swallowed air.

   F. Try simethicone (Mylicon®) drops in a dose of 0.6 ml, within 10 minutes after every feeding, for very gassy babies. Mylicon® is a very gentle antacid and anti-gas medication available over-the-counter. A dosing dropper is included. Mylicon® is safe and can be very effective in soothing colic when given as needed up to several times per day.

   G. Pay careful attention to burping your baby after feedings. Remember that you should be able to produce a burp within 2 to 3 minutes. If you cannot, stop trying. Persistent attempts may actually generate more air bubbles in your baby's stomach, thus worsening the problem. It is also possible that a silent burp of air occurred during your efforts. At this point, simply prop your baby up for more comfort. You may also try burping your baby again after 30 minutes in an upright position.

H. If your health-care provider believes that the colic is because of "reflux," a specific anti-reflux medication may be prescribed. If this does not work, your health-care provider may send you to a pediatric gastrointestinal specialist for further evaluation. This will require a comprehensive discussion with your health-care provider.

I. Keep your baby upright as much as possible after feedings. A 15- to 20-degree angle is best. This angle helps keep formula or breast milk from passively moving back up the esophagus because the food now must travel "uphill" to do so.

J. Limit the amount of time at the breast to about 10 minutes per breast, with burping in between breasts. Additional feeding time may cause more air to be swallowed.

K. If your baby is spitting up, you may be overfeeding him. Try dropping back to fewer minutes at the breast or an ounce less of formula. If you are concerned that he is not getting enough to eat, schedule a weight check with your health-care provider.

L. Try any of the additional measures below for Type 2 colic.

2. For those babies whose fussing appears to result from overstimulation (See Type 2 colic described above), you may try the following:

A. Any of the above measures for Type 1 colic.

B. While walking your baby, use the "colic hold" with baby face down, chest and shoulders on your palm, abdomen against your forearm, and legs draped over either side of your elbow.

C. Use "white noise" (for example, radio static, vacuum hum) to drown out background stimulation. You may record up to an hour of white noise on a cassette. Some babies respond to the recorded sound of a heartbeat, quiet classical music, or the gentle sound of waves.*

D. Soothing rhythmic movements: for example, rocking in arms, cradle, swing, or rocking chair.*

E. Walks in a stroller or car rides.

F. Swaddle snugly in a blanket or chest carrier, or find other ways to provide a quiet, warm, and confined environment.*

G. Pacifier to satisfy sucking need if your baby has already been recently fed and is still fussy or rooting (making sucking movements).

H. Obtain a relief caretaker for yourself for an hour or two each day, if possible. This is probably the most important way to help you and your baby!

I. A soothing, warm bath may help. Try one for baby and one for mom!

J. Try a gentle massage of your baby's tummy and thighs with a mild lotion or massage oil in light, circular, clockwise motions. You might even want to take an infant massage class.

K. Some babies are "overheated," so try unbundling your infant and see if that helps.

L. Take note of what causes increased crying in your infant. Did you go somewhere your child was overstimulated? Even if your baby slept through the experience, crying later in the day can be related to intense stimulation earlier that day.

M. Sometimes your baby simply needs to cry. If all needs have been tended to, and you are reassured that your baby is healthy, and no intervention helps, allow the baby to "have a cry" for several minutes. Some babies will self-soothe by crying. The only outcome may be a hoarse voice.

N. Make sure that you are getting a break from child care on a regular basis. This is important because it will renew and refresh you as well as give you a fresh perspective on your situation and how much you really love your baby, even though you might be very frustrated with his needs right now.

*NOTE: There are many different products at baby stores and on the Internet which are designed to accomplish these goals. They are designed for convenience but are not necessarily better than old-fashioned methods. In our opinion, whatever works best is what is best for you and your baby.

 ## Integrated Therapies

(Please refer to the section on "Administering Integrated Treatments" on page 19 for guidance on using any of the therapies that follow.)

AROMATHERAPY

• Add 1 to 2 drops of essential oil of Roman chamomile to 1 tablespoon of a carrier oil in the palm of your hand and then gently massage this onto the baby's tummy.

HERBAL REMEDIES (For quick reference please refer to the "Herbal Remedies List" on page 31 and the inside cover.)

• Beverage strength chamomile, mint, or Sleepy Time® teas brewed according to package directions (sweetened only if necessary with 1 tsp. sugar to 4 ounces of tea) may be offered in 1/2 to 2-ounce amounts several times per day (with a daily maximum of 4 ounces).

- "Gripe water" contains the herbs fennel and ginger in a solution of water with bicarbonate of soda. It often provides soothing relief for colic and is safe to use. For dosing, follow the package labeling accurately.

HOMEOPATHIC REMEDIES (For quick reference please refer to the "Homeopathic Remedies List" on page 32 and the inside cover.)

- A homeopathic remedy designed to have a soothing effect on abdominal cramping may be useful. It can be given 3 to 4 times per day as needed for relief of cramping until the colic is outgrown. (Pain 1)
- A homeopathic remedy designed to relieve the symptoms of colic may be useful. It may be given 3 to 4 times per day when your infant is not symptomatic and as often as every 15 minutes for 4 doses when colic is active. It may be used until the colic is outgrown. (Digestive 1)
- A homeopathic remedy designed to have a soothing effect on a restless infant may be useful. It can be given 3 to 6 times per day. It may be used until the colic is outgrown. (Pain 2)

BACH FLOWER REMEDIES

- Rescue Remedy™ may be of use if your child is uncomfortable from the illness, stress, or anxiety. You may use 2 drops every 10 minutes to every few hours to calm restlessness as needed.
- A lukewarm bath with 10 drops of Rescue Remedy™ added to the bathwater is often very effective at relieving agitation and stress in general.

NUTRITIONALS AND SUPPLEMENTS

- Acidophilus (baby-specific product) may be helpful, especially if mother received antibiotics during the pregnancy or while breast-feeding or if the infant has received antibiotics.

DIETARY GUIDELINES

- Sometimes colic is caused by something in a breast-feeding mother's diet. The most common foods that may cause or worsen colic are dairy foods, chocolate, gas-producing vegetables (for example, cabbage, broccoli, cauliflower, onion, garlic, and peppers), beans, spicy foods, caffeine, and anything with which you can see a "cause and effect" relationship. Occasionally, iron supplementation or prenatal vitamins with iron in the mother's diet will cause colic in the infant.

COLIC AND THE FUSSY BABY

 ## When to Call Your Health-care Provider

Call immediately if any of the following occur:
- The colic is not improved even with the above measures. That is, your baby is truly inconsolable after 2 to 3 hours of your best efforts.
- Your baby has significant vomiting, changes in bowel habits, or a distended abdomen.
- Your baby has a rectal temperature over 100 degrees and is less than 2 months old.
- You are having increasing difficulty coping with your child's colic or you are afraid you might hurt your baby.

Call within 24 hours if:
- Above measures are not helping.
- Your child has diarrhea, constipation, increased vomiting, or any other worrisome new symptoms.
- You want to check out additional treatment options not mentioned above.
- You need reassurance that your baby is "healthy," and that there are no other serious underlying problems causing so much crying.

 ## Other Relevant Sections

Abdominal Pain

Constipation

Vomiting

 ## Prevention

Prevention techniques are discussed above. Once it is clear that your child has colic, you will likely employ many of the options above in advance of the time periods you will come to know as colicky hours for your baby.

We recommend that you keep a log of your child's behaviors as this may give you clues to the most obvious causes of colic. You will begin to notice timing or feeding patterns emerge, and this predictability can help you plan ahead to avert some or all of the colic's intensity.

Conjunctivitis refers to any inflammation of the conjunctiva, which is the clear, protective tissue that covers the "whites" of the eye and the inner lining of the upper and lower eyelids. The term "pinkeye" can be used interchangeably with conjunctivitis. There are many causes of conjunctivitis, as noted below.

We have written two separate sections that describe conjunctivitis with pus and conjunctivitis without pus. Conjunctivitis with pus is most commonly associated with a bacterial infection that causes inflammation of the conjunctiva along with production of a mucous and pus discharge. The majority of other causes, including chemical, allergic, viral, and foreign body triggers, are discussed as conjunctivitis without pus.

PINKEYE, or Conjunctivitis, with Pus (EYE INFLAMMATION WITH PUS)

 ### Description/Physiology

There are many causes of pinkeye, or conjunctivitis. Pinkeye can be caused by a virus, bacteria, chemical irritant, foreign body, allergies, or trauma. When pinkeye is caused by a bacterial infection, it is usually accompanied by drainage or pus from the eye. Please see "Pinkeye Without Pus" in the next section for a discussion of the many other causes of a pinkeye/conjunctivitis infection.

Bacterial conjunctivitis is a very common infection in childhood and is definitely contagious, which makes it a source of concern to parents, schools, and daycare centers alike. It is characterized by varying degrees of redness or pinkness of the clear membrane (conjunctiva) that covers the white part of the eye and inner eyelids, and is associated with a thick, yellow discharge in the eye. The eyelids may be a bit swollen, red-rimmed, and stuck together with dried pus. Pus may accumulate as often as every 1 to 2 hours or more. The yellow crust that forms naturally during sleep is not the pus of bacterial conjunctivitis.

The bacteria reach the eye by direct contact with contaminated secretions from an infected person and will cause irritation of the conjunctiva within 3 or 4 days of exposure. In addition, mucous production is triggered by the invading bacteria.

 ### Causes/Epidemiology

There are a number of bacteria that can invade the moist membranes that protect the eye. Bacterial conjunctivitis can occur at any age.

Bacterial conjunctivitis can be seen as early as the newborn period when an

CONJUNCTIVITIS (PINKEYE)

infant is exposed to and can be infected with bacteria present in the birth canal.

In infancy, bacterial conjunctivitis can be triggered by a plugged nasolacrimal duct, commonly called the "tear duct." This duct is the channel that conducts tears from the eye into the nose. If the channel is blocked, tears and mucous cannot pass through the channel into the nose and thus back up into the eye. The static tears are susceptible to bacterial invasion, which sets up an infection. Several wipes per day of clear tears does not require treatment, but treatment is required if you're wiping pus or yellow mucous every 1 to 2 hours, or if there is significant inflammation.

 ## Expected Course

The expected course depends on several factors: the age of the child, the characteristics of the invading bacteria, other accompanying symptoms, and the general health of the child.

When nasolacrimal duct obstruction is a triggering cause of bacterial conjunctivitis, your health-care provider will likely treat with antibiotic eye ointment. This infection results from obstruction and can occur intermittently several times throughout infancy, but in most cases the obstruction is fully resolved by 12 months.

In older children, bacterial conjunctivitis most commonly presents as part of a cold syndrome. The eye can be red initially with scant discharge. As the infection progresses, there is the potential for a secondary bacterial infection accompanied by a dramatic increase in mucous production. True bacterial conjunctivitis also presents with swollen eyelids, puffiness around the lids, itchy eyes, red-rimmed eyelids, irritability, and occasional eye pain.

Bacterial conjunctivitis may accompany an ear infection.

 ## Contagiousness/Immunity

Bacterial conjunctivitis is very contagious and can spread easily in daycare centers and nurseries. It is spread through direct contact with the eye discharge of an infected child. Hand-to-eye contact is most common, and the bacteria directly infect the conjunctiva.

A child may develop bacterial conjunctivitis many times in his lifetime. There is no immunity conferred by prior episodes. In fact, a child may have more than one bout in the same season. It is particularly common in the winter months during the peak cold season.

Your child may return to school or daycare after 24 hours of antibiotic treatment and as soon as he is otherwise feeling better.

Home Care

The goals of treatment for bacterial conjunctivitis are relief of discomfort and itching and the prevention of its spread.

We ask you to read through the entire "Home Care" section to select those recommendations that make the most sense for your child's situation.

1. Cleaning the eye. Before putting in any eye medicine, remove all fresh or dried pus from the eyes and eyelids with a warm, wet cotton ball or washcloth. Wipe the eyes clear of pus as often as the pus accumulates.

2. Antibiotic eyedrops or ointments. Bacterial conjunctivitis should be treated with a prescription antibiotic eye preparation. The choice of whether to use antibiotic ointment or antibiotic eyedrops depends on the age of your child and your previous experience with ease of administration. There are several choices of effective antibiotics for bacterial conjunctivitis, and your health-care provider will choose one depending on prior history, drug allergies, and other existing factors.

   When your health-care provider prescribes antibiotic eyedrops, put 2 drops in the affected eye or eyes every 3 to 4 hours (unless otherwise noted) while your child is awake. Continue the drops for 2 additional days beyond when the mucous has disappeared and the eye has returned to normal.

   When your health-care provider prescribes antibiotic eye ointment, the ointment should be used 2 to 4 times daily. Continue the ointment for 2 additional days beyond when the mucous has disappeared and the eye has returned to normal. In general, you should expect to treat bacterial conjunctivitis for a course of 3 to 5 days.

   If an ear infection is also diagnosed at the same time, and your health-care provider prescribes an oral antibiotic, you generally will not need to use a topical eye antibiotic simultaneously, as the oral antibiotic will enter the child's tears all day and thus be an effective treatment.

   Massaging the eye, eyelids, or corners of the eye does not appear to offer any benefit and may be uncomfortable.

   If your child wears contact lenses, he should switch back temporarily to glasses until the treatment is completed. Be sure to carefully sterilize the contact lenses before he wears them again.

   For the teen who wears makeup, an episode of bacterial conjunctivitis generally means that her eye makeup is now contaminated. Throw it away and start over with new makeup. To prevent spreading conjunctivitis, eye makeup should not be shared.

CONJUNCTIVITIS (PINKEYE)

 Integrated Therapies

(Please refer to the section on "Administering Integrated Treatments" on page 19 for guidance on using any of the therapies that follow.)

HOMEOPATHIC REMEDIES (For quick reference please refer to the "Homeopathic Remedies List" on page 32 and the inside cover.)

- A homeopathic remedy designed to decrease inflammation and fever from infections may help prevent deterioration and improve the recovery time. It can be taken 3 to 6 times daily when the infection is active (for example, red or draining eyes, etc.). (General Support 2)
- A homeopathic remedy designed to relieve irritation and drainage from the eye may be helpful. It can be taken 2 to 6 times daily until the illness has resolved. (Respiratory 5)
- Homeopathic eyedrops designed to soothe the affected eye as well as to relieve irritation and drainage from the eye may be helpful. You may apply 2 drops to the affected eye or eyes 1 to 2 times daily until they are clear. (Respiratory 6)

NUTRITIONALS AND SUPPLEMENTS

- Vitamin C

 When to Call Your Health-care Provider

Call immediately if:

- The eyelids become very red, purple, or very swollen. This red or purple color may extend down onto the skin overlying the cheekbone. This may become an infection of the eyelid skin itself. This condition is called "periorbital cellulitis." A small amount of swelling and redness of the eyelid is expected with a typical "pinkeye."
- There is extreme eye pain, excessive tearing, and your child is unable to keep his eyelids open.
- There is blurred vision after the eye is cleared of mucous and pus.
- There has been direct trauma to the eye.

Call within 24 hours if:

- The infection is not cleared up after 7 days of treatment.

- Your child also develops an earache. See "Earache" section.
- The eyes become itchy, more red, and/or swollen after eye drops are begun. This may signal an allergic reaction to the eye antibiotic.
- Your child is younger than 1 month of age.

 Other Relevant Sections

Conjunctivitis (Pinkeye without pus)

Colds

Earache/Ear Infection

Sinus Infection

 Prevention

Pus from the eyes can be easily transmitted to other children by contaminated fingers. Very careful hand-washing is essential to reduce spread. You must be sure to wash your hands before and after applying eye drops or ointment or wiping your child's eyes. Encourage your child to wash his hands frequently during the day, too. Keep your infected child's washcloth and towel separate from those of other family members. Encourage your child not to touch or rub his eyes.

Your child may return to school 24 hours after eye antibiotics have been started. Yellow drainage may not completely disappear for 3 to 5 days. Your child, however, should not be contagious after the first day of antibiotic treatment. The red or pink part of the conjunctivitis may continue for a full week.

PINKEYE, or Conjunctivitis, without Pus (EYE INFLAMMATION WITHOUT PUS)

Pinkeye without pus (or conjunctivitis without pus) is a very common problem with children. It has many causes, and for our purposes, we refer to pinkeye without pus for all conjunctivitis except that triggered by bacteria (bacterial conjunctivitis).

A pink eye or red eye is characterized by a redness of a normally clear membrane (called the conjunctiva) that lies directly over the white part of the eye. There can be a clear, watery eye discharge, too, but little or no yellow discharge or matting of eyelids. This condition is often called "bloodshot eyes."

105

It is not the same as "bacterial conjunctivitis."

There are a number of different irritants that may cause red or pink eyes. Each triggering agent produces inflammation of the blood vessels of the conjunctiva and thus the pink appearance. As with most inflammatory reactions, the body produces a fluid to bathe it. In this case, the fluid is essentially a tearing reaction.

 ## Description/Physiology

"Pinkeye," or conjunctivitis without pus, is often triggered by a viral infection as part of a cold or upper respiratory infection. (See "Colds" section.) There are dozens of different viruses capable of producing "pinkeye."

Red or pink eyes can also be triggered by an irritant to the eye. The irritant can be virtually anything, including shampoo, cigarette smoke, chlorine from swimming pools, cleaning fumes, hairspray, sunscreen, excess sun exposure, and other chemicals. Environmental irritants such as dryness and pollution can cause pinkeye, as well. In young children, the irritation may be created when a child touches his eyes with hands contaminated by dirt, food, or soap.

Conjunctivitis without pus can also be triggered by a foreign body in the eye. These foreign bodies can be almost anything, including dust, an eyelash, or a fleck of sand. It is important to identify whether there is a foreign body present and where it is located. Sometimes foreign bodies can be easily removed, while others require help. In some instances an ophthalmologist may need to be consulted for the most difficult foreign body removals.

Occasionally, an eye irritant or excessive rubbing of an itchy eye may scratch the cornea (the clear structure that sits just above the pupil). This is called a "corneal abrasion." These children develop immediate and significant pain, excessive tearing, an inability to open the eye, and they may be extremely irritable. Call your health-care provider if this happens.

Allergies may also cause conjunctivitis without pus. There are usually additional allergic symptoms of itchy eyes and nose, rubbing of the eyes, sneezing, and scratchy throat. This may be classic "hay fever." (See "Hay Fever" section.) Pollens, dust, and animal dander (especially cat) are common allergy triggers. There may be some swelling of the eyelids and increased tearing. There is no other discharge. Children generally improve rapidly when the offending allergen is removed and treatments suggested below are begun.

An exhausted or sleep-deprived child may also develop pink or "bloodshot" eyes. This is especially true for children in dry climates.

If a secondary bacterial infection (bacterial conjunctivitis) occurs as a complication of any of the above causes, the clear eye discharge becomes increasingly yellow and the eyelashes may mat together after sleeping.

 ## Expected Course

The expected course of pinkeye depends largely on the triggering agent.

Viral conjunctivitis usually lasts as long as your child's cold (4 to 7 days). Most of the time, the pinkeye will resolve as the child's own immune system handles the general infection. A small percentage will go on to develop a secondary bacterial conjunctivitis.

Red eyes from irritants usually are relieved within 24 hours after washing out the irritating substance. Conjunctivitis without pus triggered by an allergy or foreign body is also improved within 24 hours after the offending agent is removed.

 ## Contagiousness/Immunity

When to send a child with pinkeye back to daycare/school is an important question. In general, although viral conjunctivitis is mildly contagious, if there is no heavy drainage suggesting a bacterial pinkeye, your child may return to school. Since irritants and allergies that trigger pinkeye are not contagious, your child does not need to be kept out of school if these are the causes.

 ## Home Care

The goals in treatment are to provide comfort from pain and itching and to reduce spread to others.

We ask you to read through the entire "Home Care" section first to select those recommendations that make the most sense for your child's situation.

1. For viral infections and mild chemical irritants, rinse the eyes with warm water or saline 4 to 5 times per day. Use a fresh, wet cotton ball each time. You may also irrigate the eyes with over-the-counter products as directed, if your child tolerates the treatment.

2. Eliminate the offending irritant when identified. For example, use goggles for swimming.

3. Add humidity to the environment. A humidifier or vaporizer will help.

4. For allergy triggers, remove the offending allergen. The allergen (such as dust, pollen, or makeup) should be removed from the face with thorough rinses with salt water. Be sure to wash the hair, because these allergens can cling to hair, as well. Encourage your child to avoid rubbing his eyes as much as possible.

5. Cold compresses applied to the eyelids can also be of great help.

6. If the eye remains very itchy from an allergy, you may try an OTC vasoconstrictor drop such as Visine® or Naphcon A®. Doses vary, but generally we recommend 2 to 3 drops 2 to 3 times per day. These preparations are not recommended for use over more than 5 days.

7. Finally, if that fails, you may try an oral antihistamine, such as Benadryl®. Nighttime use is always best because Benadryl® may cause drowsiness.

8. General treatment of viral respiratory symptoms may incidentally help viral pinkeye. See "Colds" section.

9. Protect the eyes from overexposure to the sun with effective sunglasses, especially on sunny days, in the snow, and at high altitude. The conjunctiva can be sunburned!

 ## Integrated Therapies

(Please refer to the section on "Administering Integrated Treatments" on page 19 for guidance on using any of the therapies that follow.)

HERBAL REMEDIES (For quick reference please refer to the "Herbal Remedies List" on page 31 and the inside cover.)

- Echinacea/astragalus can be used to support the immune system in helping to resolve a viral infection. For dosing, follow the package labeling accurately.

HOMEOPATHIC REMEDIES (For quick reference please refer to the "Homeopathic Remedies List" on page 32 and the inside cover.)

- A homeopathic remedy designed to decrease inflammation and fever from infections may help prevent deterioration and improve the recovery time. It can be taken 3 to 6 times daily when the infection is active (for example, red or draining eyes, etc.). (General Support 2)

- A homeopathic remedy designed to relieve irritation and drainage from the eye may be helpful. It can be taken 2 to 6 times daily until the illness has resolved. (Respiratory 5)

- Homeopathic eye drops designed to both soothe the affected eye and to relieve irritation and drainage from the eye may be helpful. You may apply 2 drops to the affected eye or eyes 1 to 2 times daily until they are clear. (Respiratory 6)
- A homeopathic remedy designed to help minimize the impact of allergies from any cause may be helpful when allergies are suspected. It can be taken 2 to 6 times daily during times when the eye is pink. (Respiratory 7)

NUTRITIONALS AND SUPPLEMENTS

- Vitamin C

DIETARY GUIDELINES

- Avoid any food that you know your child has allergic reactions to.

 When to Call Your Health-care Provider

Call immediately if:
- The eyelids become very red, purple, or swollen.
- There is moderate to extreme pain, excessive tearing, and inability to look toward light.
- There has been direct trauma to the eye.
- There was a chemical splashed into the eye.
- Vision is blurred.

Call within 24 hours if:
- A yellow discharge develops. See "Conjunctivitis (Pinkeye with Pus)" section.
- The redness itself lasts for more than 7 days.

 Other Relevant Sections

Conjunctivitis (Pinkeye with Pus)
Colds
Hay Fever
Sunburn

Prevention

Prevention of pinkeye without pus depends on the usual triggers. If an allergy is suspected, avoidance of the allergy triggers is important. See "Hay Fever" section.

Careful hand-washing will remove grit and grime that might accidentally be swept into the eye.

Viral infections require careful hand-washing to prevent spread. Hand-washing is important for both the care provider and the child.

Description/Physiology

Constipation is defined as: (1) a hard-textured stool or (2) a stool that is difficult or painful to pass. Acute (sudden onset) constipation is a common and often easily remedied childhood symptom. Chronic constipation is less common but more difficult to remedy, because there is often a behavioral component to the problem.

Constipation may be associated with a decrease in stool frequency; however, infrequency may also occur with a normal or even a loose stool. While constipation is often associated with infrequent stools, infrequency and constipation are separate symptoms.

It is common for infants to grunt a bit and strain during a bowel movement, and these infants may be "over-diagnosed" with constipation. Most young infants (birth to 2 months and especially those who are breast-fed) may have a bowel movement triggered by each feeding, although this "gastro-colic" reflex lessens as a child ages.

You will develop a clear sense of your child's stooling patterns within a few weeks, although for some infants, no predictable pattern may emerge.

Causes/Epidemiology

There are many, many causes of constipation that depend on the age of the child, other symptoms present, behavioral factors, and diet. The increased firmness of the stool is due to a relative lack of water in the stool. Some of the features of the two definitions of constipation listed above may occur together or separately.

Constipation is an abnormally hard stool generally caused by a relative lack of fiber and/or water in the diet. Constipation is not only uncomfortable but, when chronic, it increases the risk of many different diseases, including hemorrhoids, fissures, urinary tract infections, etc. It may also make toilet training more difficult. Thus, it is not only important to resolve constipation when it occurs but also to prevent it from becoming a chronic problem.

In older children, several additional external factors may trigger constipation, including emotional stress, transitions such as a new sibling or a move, traveling, school problems and parental pressures for toilet training, as well as too much dietary fat, too much processed food and dairy products, and not enough whole foods!

Holding back stool is common in some older children. The fear of pain, the production of blood because of a small tear (fissure), the fear of the toilet itself or having a bowel movement in a public place (such as school bathrooms) can all contribute to stool retention and cause chronic constipation. Some children will complain of a stomachache, as well. All of this can set in motion a vicious cycle of increased retention, with increased pain and the infrequent passage of a large stool, further retention, and the final production of a huge, painful stool that only reinforces the fear process all over again.

Some older children are constipated because of medications they are taking. Consult your health-care provider about possible constipating side effects of medicine.

There are many rare causes of constipation. While some parents worry about an "obstruction," it is very unlikely that an obstruction has occurred unless your child has severe, abrupt pain with abdominal distension and vomiting. These children are generally very ill.

Toilet training is an entirely different subject that requires special attention and specific approaches. This discussion is beyond the scope of this handbook. For further guidance you may want to consult your health-care provider.

Constipation is not stool infrequency. Stool infrequency—stools of normal consistency but few in number—is especially common in infants who are breast-fed. It occurs most often during the second month of life and thereafter. These infants may go as long as 7 to 10 days without a stool! Infants with this infrequent stooling pattern may have a good deal of gas and are often very fussy around the time of the bowel movement. If infrequency is not associated with any other symptom, you may be sure that this is a normal stooling variation and requires no treatment. If your breast-fed baby is generally happy, growing well, and has a good appetite, there is no need to worry.

 ## Home Care

The primary goals for treatment are to provide relief of constipation, to make suggestions about prevention of future episodes, and to make your child comfortable. We ask you to first read through the entire "Home Care" section below to select those recommendations that make the most sense for your child's current situation.

1. For infants less than 6 months (in our order of preference):
   A. Try adding 2 to 3 ounces of water to your child's daily fluid intake, 1 to 2 times daily.
   B. Try a formula change. Good Start® formula may produce a softer stool in some infants. Call your health-care provider for other suggestions.

C. Add corn syrup (Karo® syrup, dark or light), 1 to 2 teaspoons per bottle of formula or pumped breast milk, with a maximum of 6 teaspoons per day. Start with the lower dose and increase by $1/2$ teaspoon increments per bottle every day until your infant is having a soft bowel movement at least daily. Do not use honey!!!

D. If the corn syrup fails to help within 4 to 5 days, discontinue it and try a "fiber source" such as Maltsupex®. The dose range for this product is $1/2$ to 2 teaspoons, 2 to 3 times per day. This is an over-the-counter preparation but needs to be special-ordered by the pharmacist.

E. If all else fails, you may consider rectal administration of one "infant" sized glycerin suppository to assist your child in having a bowel movement, while you continue to use steps A through D above. You should call your health-care provider if glycerin suppositories are required more than one time or do not work. Glycerin suppositories, once started, are generally used daily for up to 10 days until he has a daily BM on his own.

F. Gentle massage of your infant's lower abdomen may help.

2. For infants and children older than 6 months, use any of the preventive measures listed above, and you may also try the following:

A. Give fruit juices (such as apple, grape, prune); 2 to 4 ounces per day may be sufficient. Undiluted juices are better laxatives than diluted juices, but for infants 6 to 12 months of age, start with diluted or "baby" prune juice first. Good old prune juice often does the trick! Whole fruits like pears and prunes provide a great fiber source for infants older than 6 months.

B. Maltsupex® or Metamucil® in a dose of $1/2$ to 2 teaspoons given 2 to 3 times per day. Begin with a low dose (for example, $1/2$ teaspoon twice daily) and increase by $1/2$ teaspoon increments every day until your child passes a normal, soft stool daily. Fiber supplements must be accompanied by increased water or juice to be effective.

C. Do not use adult laxatives, mineral oil, cathartics, suppositories, or enemas without calling your health-care provider first. They may prescribe Milk of Magnesia® as one example. Certainly no laxative should be used for more than a few days without your health-care provider's direction. In the same way, mineral oil, used over a long period of time, may cause problems, including leakage and vitamin malabsorption. Glycerin suppositories may be used also, but you should call if they are required more than one time or do not work.

113

D. Consider using oat (refortified) cereal instead of rice cereal, if your infant becomes constipated.

E. Increase other fiber sources in your child's diet. Fruits such as apple, orange, pear, or prune may initially be sufficient. Vegetables and bran, and products with bran, are good sources of constipation relief. Popcorn is an excellent fiber source for children over 5 years of age. Dark, leafy vegetables rich in magnesium may also help. Dairy can be very constipating, so please limit milk and cheese intake. Bananas and cooked carrots can also be constipating and are best avoided in general.

F. For your older child, train him to sit on the potty after meals. This is the time when the entire digestive system is "revved up," and your child can begin to sense the push of stool triggered by the meal. Five minutes on the potty after meals for several days in a row may help establish a regular pattern of stooling. Try a sticker chart to reward successful daily bowel movements.

G. If stool gets "stuck" in the anal canal, you may need to help relieve the blockage. This can be done by gentle traction on the stool, lubrication, and rectal stimulation around the anal sphincter with a finger lubricated with petroleum jelly.

H. Older children may experience leakage of softer stool around a large, hard plug of stool collected in the lower colon. This may manifest as frequent soiling in the underwear of small amounts of stool. Call your health-care provider if that happens and appears to have become a chronic problem.

I. If a red ring forms around the anus, you may apply Lotrimin® cream or Neosporin Ointment® liberally on the inflamed tissue. This will help control yeast and/or bacterial production in this area as well as provide some lubrication to facilitate stool passage.

J. If your child is complaining of anal area pain while attempting to have a stool, an application of Neosporin Plus® will help temporarily numb the area, permitting a less painful experience for him.

 ## Integrated Therapies

(Please refer to the section on "Administering Integrated Treatments" on page 19 for guidance on using any of the therapies that follow.)

AROMATHERAPY

- An aromatherapy bath or massage with the essential oil lavender can soothe and relax your child's anxiety and restlessness that can accompany constipation. Add 2 to 5 drops of oil to a warm bath and allow your child to soak for a comfortable period of time.

- If there is inflammation around the anus associated with constipation, add 1 to 2 drops each of the essentials oils of German chamomile and lavender to 1 ounce of carrier oil and mix well. Then gently massage around the anus twice daily to soothe the pain and discomfort.

HERBAL REMEDIES (For quick reference please refer to the "Herbal Remedies List" on page 31 and the inside cover.)

- Aloe vera juice (food grade) may help with chronic constipation. You may have to give it with juice to improve its flavor. Start with a dose of 1 tbsp. twice daily and increase by 1 tbsp. increments every 5 to 7 days to a maximum dose of 2 ounces twice a day.

HOMEOPATHIC REMEDIES (For quick reference please refer to the "Homeopathic Remedies List" on page 32 and the inside cover.)

- A homeopathic remedy designed to promote bowel movement regularity may be helpful for chronic constipation. It may be given 2 to 3 times a day for long periods of time. (Digestive 2)

BACH FLOWER REMEDIES

- Rescue Remedy™ may be of use if your child is uncomfortable from the illness, stress, or anxiety. You may use 2 drops every 10 minutes to every few hours to calm restlessness as needed.
- Vine, Vervain, Chestnut Budd, Mimulus, and Rock Rose may be of help in the chronically constipated child who is stubborn and/or afraid of using the toilet. (You may wish to consult your health-care provider on how to mix and dose these remedies.)

NUTRITIONALS AND SUPPLEMENTS

- Magnesium
- EFAs
- Probiotics

DIETARY GUIDELINES

- Fiber and water are the two most important dietary ingredients to improve chronic constipation. There are a wide variety of fiber supplements available and the most important feature is that it tastes good, since it is likely that your child will need to take it for a long time. You may give 3 to 8 grams of dietary fiber (read the nutritional panel to determine the amount of fiber in your product) with 6 to 8 ounces of water or juice twice per day. DO NOT GIVE THE FIBER WITHOUT THE FLUID, AS FIBER WHEN GIVEN ALONE CAN HARDEN STOOL.

• Prunes as fruit or juice can be used and the amount should be adjusted based on what is effective. With infants and toddlers you may begin with 1/2 to 1 ounce 2 to 3 times daily and increase from there.

• Avoid foods that are known to be constipating, such as dairy products, bananas, apples (juice is OK), rice, cooked carrots, and toasted foods.

• Encourage foods that tend to soften stool, such as cooked and raw fruits, vegetables, high-fiber cereals, and grains. Mix a high-fiber cereal with their favorite cereal in the morning.

 ## When to Call Your Health-care Provider

Constipation is rarely an emergency. Your call can generally wait until morning.

Call immediately if:
• Your child is straining to have a bowel movement with inconsolable pain for longer than 30 to 60 minutes.
• Your child refuses to nurse for several hours beyond regular feeding time. See "Dehydration" section.
• You see a large amount of blood in the stool.
• Your child complains of significant and worsening abdominal pain.
• You cannot extract an impacted stool after an hour of trying and your child is very uncomfortable.

Call within 24 hours if:
• The above measures do not work.
• A small amount of blood appears in or on the stool.
• Mild to moderate abdominal pain or excessive gas develops.
• Your child appears to be avoiding bowel movements by willfully holding them.
• Your infant has not had a bowel movement in ten days (if breast-fed), in spite of the above measures.
• Your older child has not had a bowel movement in three days in spite of the above measures.

- You feel that you must try a suppository, enema, cathartic, or mineral oil.
- There is a worsening area of redness around the anus in spite of above treatments.
- Your infant is less than 14 days of age and has not had a bowel movement in the past 48 hours.

Other Relevant Sections

Abdominal Pain

Dehydration

Diarrhea

Prevention

Many general principles for prevention are discussed above. In addition, you may try the following:

1. Improve dietary fiber intake by increasing foods that are high in fiber—vegetables, fruits, grains, beans, and nuts; and decreasing foods that have no fiber—meat, poultry, fish, dairy products, and eggs.
2. Avoid foods that are known to be constipating, such as dairy products, bananas, rice, processed foods, and toasted foods (crackers).
3. Maintain good daily fluid intake. Have a water bottle easily accessible at all times.
4. Addition of a daily "fiber supplement" in a dose of 5 to 10 grams, with 8 to 20 ounces of extra fluid per day, may be required. (Please consult your health-care provider if you feel that this step is necessary.)
5. Prunes or prune juice (undiluted) given daily may prevent constipation.
6. Increasing your child's activity can help, especially if he hasn't been getting regular exercise.

Description/Physiology

A cough is caused by an irritation of the airway or lungs. It may serve as a natural, protective reflex to prevent mucous from accumulating in the airways as well as to expel bacteria, viruses, allergens, chemical toxins, and other irritants out of the lungs.

The cough itself can present with all types of characteristics. It can be harsh, hacking, wet, mucousy, high-pitched, gasping, or barking. The quality of the cough is helpful in the diagnosis of its cause. Listening to the cough over the phone or during an office examination may be a useful tool for evaluation.

Coughing can also be exhausting and often disrupts sleep. Sleep deprivation slows healing, so special attention should be paid to the nighttime cough. In general, it is best to allow the discharge and movement of mucous out of the airway via a strong cough, but at night, sleep becomes the top priority.

Some coughs are so strong that they precipitate a vomiting episode. While this is an unpleasant event, it is not dangerous, and the vomiting due to coughing may serve to clear the digestive tract of swallowed mucous. Persistent vomiting must be evaluated, however.

Causes/Epidemiology

Coughing is associated with several illnesses, the most common of which are simple upper respiratory infections (colds) and allergies. These children are usually not very ill. See "Cold" section and "Hay Fever" section. Other less common causes of coughing include pneumonia, asthma, croup, bronchitis, bronchiolitis, and a foreign body in the airway. These sources of coughing are usually associated with a more ill-appearing child who has more worrisome symptoms: high fever, increased breathing rate, lethargy, dehydration, labored respirations, and usually a more severe cough.

Allergy, sinus infection, chemical irritation (such as smoke), or dry irritation of the back of the throat may cause a dry, hacking, tickle-triggered cough. A postnasal drip of mucous from congested sinuses and an inflamed nose from colds, flu, sinus infections, etc., tend to cause a cough that is worse at night when your child is lying down. There is often an accompanying clear runny nose, itchy eyes, and sneezing with allergies.

Coughing may also be a sign of a primary lung problem in the lower tracts of the lung. If a cough accompanies a rapid rate of breathing along with a fever in an ill-looking child, pneumonia may be present. Children with asthma usually have a cough accompanied by wheezing triggered by bronchospasm (acute narrowing of the airways). See "Asthma" section.

Younger children may inhale small objects, such as toys, peanuts, and popcorn into their airway (aspiration). These aspirations often produce immediate symptoms such as choking and labored breathing, but, alternatively, may only produce a chronic cough and minimal wheezing. Rapid progression of severe respiratory distress in a small child is often caused by an aspiration. If the airway is completely obstructed, this is an absolute medical emergency. Your child may be unable to cry or speak, appear frantic, turn blue, and eventually lose consciousness. This is clearly a 911 call! See "Choking" section in First Aid.

Croup has a unique cough that sounds like a "barking seal." Also, your child may have very labored inspiration (breathing in) that is called "stridor," exaggerated chest movements, and obvious distress. See "Croup" section.

If your child has not been vaccinated against pertussis (whooping cough) or is an older child whose vaccine has "worn off," it is possible that pertussis is the causative agent. The classical cough of pertussis is a harsh, staccato series of coughs ending in a loud, inspiratory "whoop." However, pertussis can mimic other coughs such as the "barking cough" of croup.

Coughs may also be triggered by exercise. We most commonly think of exercise-induced asthma when this happens. See "Asthma" section.

In some instances, the mere act of exercising, especially in cold or polluted air, may trigger a cough when there is no actual wheezing and a child is not an asthmatic.

 Expected Course

A cough usually lasts for several days until the other symptoms of an upper respiratory infection resolve. However, a cough may persist for up to 4 to 6 weeks following any acute respiratory illness, while the body's own immune system works to clear the airways of inflammation and mucous debris. This lingering cough is often referred to as a "post-infectious cough," because there is no longer any active virus or bacteria present, but airway irritation remains.

A chronic cough, lasting several weeks and without an improving response to the usual relief methods listed below, warrants attention. Common causes of chronic cough include sinus disease, asthma, and allergies. The full evaluation of a chronic cough may include a chest x-ray, blood work, or special lung function testing. In some cases, your health-care provider may recommend further evaluation by a lung specialist, allergist, or ear, nose, and throat (ENT) doctor.

Contagiousness/Immunity

The contagiousness of a cough depends on its trigger. Many viral causes are easily transmitted in the air by the cough to another child or adult. Direct contact with oral and nasal secretions is the most common mode of transmission of a virus. Bacterial transmission through the air is also possible, though less common.

 ## Home Care

The goals of treatment for a cough are relief of discomfort from the cough itself, preservation of sleep, prevention of spread of an infectious trigger, and return to normal activity. We ask you to first read through the entire "Home Care" section and select those recommendations that make the most sense for your child's current symptoms.

1. Decrease mucous thickness and production by the following means:
   A. Encourage intake of clear liquids (Water, Pedialyte®, Jell-O® water, and Sleepytime® tea). Warm liquids help relax the airway and loosen mucous. You may also try warm apple juice, lemonade, or warm tea. Milk, formula, and other dairy products are mucous-producing and should be avoided if at all possible. This may, of course, be difficult in very small infants who are only breast- or formula-fed. In general, breast-feeding should not be interrupted, but shorter, more frequent breast feedings may be easier for your infant. Use your best judgment. Hydration is essential to mobilize mucous, bacteria, viruses, and other irritants from the airways.
   B. Use a cool-mist or steam humidifier or vaporizer in your child's bedroom and/or play area. You need not add medication to the water. Be very careful about following the manufacturers' instructions about frequent cleaning to avoid buildup of chemical or mold irritants. (NOTE: Always monitor your child when using steam to avoid accidental burns.)
   C. Decongestant preparations are generally discouraged, as they thicken the mucous instead of allowing it to drain effectively. Your child may have short-term, immediate relief with these medications, but in the long run these drugs may actually thicken mucous enough to lead to a secondary bacterial infection, such as a sinus infection or ear infection, if this thick mucous does not drain.

D. Elevate the head of the bed to roughly a 10-degree angle. This can be accomplished by placing pillows or rolled towels under the mattress. Of course, the restless child may end up in all sorts of positions at night, but give it a try!

E. If the above measures do not produce improvement, try placing your child in a steamy bathroom (similar to treatment for croup) for 20 to 30 minutes, especially during cough spasms. This high concentration of humidification may help shrink swollen tissues or coat a dry throat, or loosen nasal or sinus mucous.

2. Use cough suppressants only if the cough is interfering with your child's sleep, school attendance, or other important daily activities. We prefer to limit cough suppressants to nighttime use only, but we realize that some daytime activities can be disrupted by an incessant coughing. Suppressants include:

A. Corn syrup (for children under 1 year of age) or honey (only for children over 1 year of age) mixed with lemon juice in warm liquid or tea (especially Throat Coat® by Traditional Medicinals) will soothe a sore throat and decrease an irritating cough.

B. A cough preparation containing dextromethorphan, such as Delsym®, is most effective. This is an over-the-counter preparation. Please see "OTC Medication Recommendations and Dosages" section.

C. Most coughs in children over 4 years of age may be controlled by cough drops sucked often.

D. Codeine is rarely more effective than OTC preparations and should be used only on your health-care provider's recommendation. Codeine preparations are available only by prescription.

E. Expectorants (such as guainfenesin) are generally of minimal value.

3. Do not let anyone smoke around your coughing child. This includes smoke in the air as well as smoke infused into clothing. Teenagers should be warned against smoking during an illness and counseled about stopping smoking altogether.

A. Outside activity should be restricted as the cough worsens. Cold air, air pollution, and air breathed during high allergy seasons are common cough triggers.

B. Herbal chest rubs may help. Vicks Vaporub® is fine, too.

Integrated Therapies

(Please refer to the section on "Administering Integrated Treatments" on page 19 for guidance on using any of the therapies that follow.)

AROMATHERAPY

- Add 2 drops each of the essential oils of eucalyptus radiata and lavender to 1 to 2 teaspoons of olive oil and rub on your child's chest to soothe a cough or congestion.
- An aromatherapy bath or massage with the essential oils of eucalyptus radiata and/or lavender can soothe and relax your child's anxiety and restlessness as well as his congestion and difficult breathing. Add 2 to 5 drops of oil to a warm bath and allow your child to soak for a comfortable period of time.

HERBAL REMEDIES (For quick reference please refer to the "Herbal Remedies List" on page 31 and the inside cover.)

- Horehound may be very effective in reducing mucous production and thus improves a wet cough. It may help in the recuperative phase of a cough, if there is a significant amount of mucous production. For dosing, follow the package labeling accurately.
- Cherry bark may be very effective in reducing the duration of a dry, irritant cough. For dosing, follow the package labeling accurately.
- Valerian root is a mild herbal sedative that may offer some help in easing a child with a significant cough. Valerian root may be most useful at bedtime. For dosing, follow the package labeling accurately.
- Herbal teas may offer some soothing relief of cold symptoms and also provide a good source of fluids. Herb teas made from Chamomile or Mint as well as a variety of blended herbal teas (refer to "Herbal Therapies" section) can be brewed according to package directions, sweetened to taste, and offered frequently throughout the day.

HOMEOPATHIC REMEDIES (For quick reference please refer to the "Homeopathic Remedies List" on page 32 and the inside cover.)

- A homeopathic remedy designed to reduce the cough reflex and irritation may be helpful in shortening the duration of the cough. It can be given 2 to 3 times per day until the cough subsides or resolves. (Respiratory 8)
- A homeopathic remedy designed to decrease inflammation from infections or other irritants may help prevent deterioration and

improve the recovery time. It can be taken 3 to 6 times daily for several weeks as long as the cough is improving. (General Support 2)

BACH FLOWER REMEDIES

- Rescue Remedy™ may be of use if your child has anxiety with episodes of coughing. You may use 2 drops every 10 minutes to every few hours to calm restlessness as needed.

NUTRITIONALS AND SUPPLEMENTS

- Vitamin A
- Vitamin C

DIETARY GUIDELINES

- Avoid mucous-forming foods, especially all dairy products and citrus fruits and their juices.
- Warm foods (soup) and beverages (tea) can often provide temporary relief from a cough.

INTEGRATIVE SUPPORTIVE CARE

- Please read the section "Integrated Management of Respiratory Illnesses."

 When to Call Your Health-care Provider

Call immediately if any of the following occur:
- Shortness of breath or rapid breathing rate (over 50 to 60 breaths per minute in an infant or over 40 breaths per minute in children over the age of 2 years), especially in the absence of fever.
- Blueness of lips or fingernails.
- Long pauses between breaths (more than 5 to 10 seconds) in infants.
- Spasms that cause choking, passing out, or persistent vomiting.
- Blood coughed up in sputum or mucous.
- Vomiting blood.
- Sudden onset of violent coughing in a child who might have aspirated a small object.
- Wheezing that is worsening.
- Increased work of breathing with heaving respirations and deep up-and-down chest wall excursions.

COUGH

- Stridor (harsh inspiratory breathing; see "Croup" section) develops that does not respond to our croup recommendations.
- Rapid onset of sharp and persistent chest pain.
- Increasing lethargy.
- Signs of increasing dehydration. See "Dehydration" section.

Call within 24 hours if:
- Mild wheezing is not gone in 24 hours.
- Croupy, "barking seal" type cough with any difficulty in breathing develops.
- There is sustained increase above normal respiratory rate for 6 hours.
- Fever lasts more than 72 hours.
- Child less than 3 months has a cough lasting over 48 hours.
- Cough produces yellow-green discharge.
- Chest pain occurs in older children.
- You think your child has a "whooping" cough and may have pertussis, especially if unimmunized.
- Cough lasts over 2 weeks.
- Cough interferes with sleep or causes several days of missed school.

Other Relevant Sections

Asthma
Bronchiolitis
Bronchitis
Colds
Croup
Dehydration
Sinus Infection
Throat
First Aid—Choking
Integrated Management of Respiratory Illnesses

Prevention

To help prevent the spread of an infectious cough, teach your child to cough into his arm or sleeve rather than into a hand that is sure to touch many other sites. Cough prevention is a function of addressing the exact trigger of the cough. Please refer to the appropriate sections of illnesses in which cough is a prominent element for the prevention tips specific to that trigger. In addition, many of the suggestions for care listed above can be converted to useful prevention techniques.

CROUP

 Description/Physiology

Croup can be one of the most frightening respiratory illnesses of childhood. The signs and symptoms of croup may vary, depending on the child and the child's age, but the common ones are as follows:

- Fever—ranges from 99 to 105 degrees, usually 101 to 103 degrees. See "Fever" section.
- Irritability—children are cranky and uncomfortable, especially when the temperature is elevated or if they are frightened.
- Sore throat—older children may complain of sore throats, and younger babies may simply refuse to drink, put their fingers in their mouth, or drool even more than usual. See "Sore Throat" section.
- Cold symptoms—
  - Runny nose, usually clear and moderate amounts.
  - Cough—characteristically a "barking seal" cough, can be very severe and spasmodic, especially bad at night, and difficult to suppress.
  - Red eyes—especially when temperature is elevated. Rarely is pinkeye with pus present. See "Cold," "Cough," and "Pinkeye" sections.
- Poor appetite and decrease in fluid intake—because of sore throat, disinterest, and general achiness.
- Voice changes and/or loss of voice—because of swelling in and around the vocal cords.
- Finally, and most worrisome, is stridor. Stridor is a harsh, inspiratory (breathing in) sound, often accompanied by anxiety and increased work of breathing. Stridor is the result of a narrowing of the opening to the vocal cords because of inflammation and mucous. Stridor often begins abruptly in the middle of the night with a child who has had cold symptoms for a day or two.

In some cases, stridor is the first symptom to present in a previously healthy child. This is particularly frightening. In this instance, parents might think their child has aspirated (choked on) an object. Parents also worry that the child could stop breathing altogether. This is very, very unlikely to ever happen.

Croup with stridor requires a doctor's attention and may even require hospitalization if not resolved. Stridor typically occurs at night. Stridor during daylight hours is a warning that particularly bad stridor could occur after nightfall and that a difficult night may lie ahead.

Many children with croup have the "crowing" sound (stridor) only when upset, crying, and/or anxious. Children with more severe cases will have stridor while at rest, made even worse with crying. In some children the muscles between the ribs or in the neck may pull in with each inspiration. These movements are called "retractions" and are a sign of worsening respiratory distress.

In older children, whom you think should have outgrown croup by now, croup can be particularly frightening. Stridor in a 10-year-old is also often abrupt in onset, can be severe, and can produce considerable anxiety in the child.

Causes/Epidemiology

Croup is a very common respiratory problem in children in dry climates. It can affect children of all ages, from newborns to children as old as 10 years, but it is predominantly found in the 6-month through 4-year-old age group. Croup is commonly a fall and winter disease, and while we see it as early as September, we may also see it as late as May and even sporadically over the summer.

Classic croup is most frequently caused by a virus called the parainfluenza virus. As the name of the virus suggests, it is similar to the influenza virus, which is the cause of the "flu."

Less common causes of croup may include other respiratory viruses, some bacteria, aspirating a foreign body into an airway, and even allergies. They can produce a "croup-like syndrome" indistinguishable from the croup caused by parainfluenza virus. Epiglottitis is another cause of stridor that is generally caused by bacteria we can now prevent through childhood immunizations. Swelling of the epiglottis, which is the protective "flap" over the upper airway, is characterized by severe drooling of all airway secretions, little or no cough, and high fever, and often the child will lean forward to help keep the airway open. Epiglottitis is a rapidly progressive, life-threatening, swelling of the airway. You should call your health-care provider immediately if you suspect its presence, especially in an un-immunized child.

Stridor can also occur from an insect sting or after an allergenic food, which triggers a severe allergic reaction, is ingested. You may observe hives and swelling of the face and neck, as well. While this is unlikely, it is a severe allergic reaction, called anaphylaxis. Anaphylaxis is a life-threatening emergency; dial 911 immediately. Do not waste precious time calling your health-care provider.

Children can have croup more than one time in a single winter season. In fact, some children can have multiple bouts of croup in a given year. When there is recurrent croup, your health-care provider may consult with an ear, nose, and throat (ENT) doctor to be certain there is not an anatomical abnormality which further predisposes your child to repeated bouts of croup. This may involve the ENT doctor's directly examining the throat and larynx. On occasion, a vocal cord abnormality is discovered.

 ## Contagiousness/Immunity

Croup is spread most easily through nasal and oral secretions. Sharing recently contaminated utensils, toys, cups, towels, etc., can also spread the virus. This is why careful hand-washing is essential to prevent the spread of croup. This is especially true when newborns, the elderly, or chronically ill children are involved. The virus can also be transmitted through the air by a forceful, barky cough when tiny mucous droplets are expelled into the air.

Why some children develop croup and stridor when exposed to the croup virus while other children do not, depends on the child's immune system and the airway anatomy. The soft airway tissues in some children are simply more susceptible to the swelling and subsequent narrowing triggered by the virus than in other children.

Your child is contagious approximately two days before major croup symptoms develop. During that time, the developing cold symptoms produce mucous with a very high concentration of virus present. The point at which your child is no longer contagious is difficult to know precisely. Certainly, your child is contagious during the fever phase, but is less so as symptoms improve. Your child is safe to return to daycare or school 48 hours after the fever has gone and when symptoms are considerably improved.

 ## Home Care

The treatment goals are to relieve discomfort, improve hydration, preserve sleep, reduce spread of the virus, and return your child to normal activity as soon as possible. We ask you to first read the entire "Home Care" section to determine which of our recommendations make the most sense for your child's current symptoms.

The mainstays of home therapy are as follows:

1. Keep your child as calm as possible. Croup is a frightening experience for a child, so your immediate, nurturing attention will reduce anxiety and ease respiratory distress. Your child will react to your own anxiety with further fear and agitation. You may feel more comfortable sleeping in your child's room for a night or two!

2. Humidification—for all degrees of croup, mild to severe, we recommend that you run a vaporizer or humidifier (preferably cold, but hot is fine) continuously in your child's bedroom and play area. You may spread a wet sheet, partially covering the crib or draped like a tent over the bed, with the steam pumped directly into this "croup tent."

3. To relieve stridor, very effective humidification can also be achieved by steam from a hot shower. Place your child in a steamy bathroom for 15 to 20 minutes or until the stridor is relieved. Continue to calm your child by cuddling or reading a story. There may be resistance initially to the steamy bathroom, but your reassurance and calm manner can relieve that anxiety. Then, return your child to his bedroom with the humidifier on full blast!

4. If the steamy bathroom fails to relieve stridor, bundle your child up very warmly and accompany him outside into the cold evening air (garage or backyard). This cold air helps shrink swollen throat tissues very effectively. If there is definite benefit within 10 minutes, you should remain outside another 10 to 15 minutes to fully interrupt this stridor cycle. The colder the air, the better it is. It is critical that your child not get chilled as this can cause agitation and worsen the stridor—so keep them bundled up. We know it seems contradictory to take a sick child outside into the cold air, but it works! Here is one very common middle-of-the-night example: A child awakens with stridor, parents panic, and they rush the child to the emergency room. En route, the child breathes the cold night air, and arrives at the ER perfectly fine.

You may have to alternate the cold air outside with the steamy bathroom inside 1 or 2 times each to break the stridor. Doing so might avoid a visit to an emergency room. Once the stridor has been interrupted, you can see your health-care provider the next morning. If stridor persists or recurs in spite of these measures, your health-care provider should be called at that time.

Most children will eventually calm down and sleep through the remainder of the night. Even if your child does so and awakens the next morning with only cold symptoms remaining, but no stridor, please call your health-care provider for further instructions. Our experience is that one night of stridor means that a second, even worse one may be coming. There are measures your health-care provider can take after they have examined your child that can make the second and third nights stridor-free.

5. Other helpful measures include the following:
    A. Give acetaminophen or ibuprofen for discomfort of fever, especially if the fever exceeds 103 degrees or causes general achiness in the older child. See

"Fever" section. (Note: Ibuprofen, with its anti-inflammatory effect, may actually help reduce the vocal cord swelling more than Tylenol®.)

B. Increase fluid intake with clear liquids while avoiding milk. Dairy products can produce mucous, which further blocks the already swollen airway. Warm teas and warm, clear soup can relax throat muscles. See "Dehydration" section.

C. Elevate the head of the bed or crib, if possible, by placing a rolled towel under the mattress, or adding a pillow for the older child. Many children with stridor prefer to be as upright as possible

D. Occasional use of a cough suppressant at night, when no other methods relieve the cough for sleeping. See "Cough" section.

E. Finally, your health-care provider may use a prescription steroid medication, Decadron®, as one last outpatient therapy to reduce stridor and hopefully prevent hospitalization. Decadron® possesses a powerful anti-inflammatory action. It causes a marked decrease in the swelling and inflammation of the vocal cord area.

   Decadron® can only be prescribed after your child's croup is confirmed by your health-care provider's examination or in the emergency room. If Decadron® fails, a hospital admission for observation and breathing treatments may be required.

F. Antibiotics are not necessary in croup since it is a viral illness, unless there is another infection (such as a bacterial ear infection) present at the same time.

G. Avoid cigarette exposure for your croupy child.

H. Avoid sedating medicines such as Benadryl®, as they may further weaken your child's respiratory drive and suppress the cough.

 Integrated Therapies

(Please refer to the section on "Administering Integrated Treatments" on page 19 for guidance on using any of the therapies that follow.)

AROMATHERAPY

* An aromatherapy bath or massage with the essential oils of eucalyptus radiata and/or lavender can soothe and relax your child's anxiety and restlessness as well as his congestion and difficult breathing. Add 2 to 5 drops of oil to a warm bath and allow your child to soak for a comfortable period of time.

- Add 2 drops each of the essential oils of eucalyptus radiata and lavender to 1 to 2 teaspoons of olive oil and rub on your child's chest to soothe a cough or congestion.
- Add 5 to 8 drops each of ravensara aromatica and frankincense (best species is boswellia carteri) to a steam humidifier at the child's bedside or in a croup tent.

HERBAL REMEDIES (For quick reference please refer to the "Herbal Remedies List" on page 31 and the inside cover.)

- Horehound may be very effective in reducing mucous production and thus improves a wet cough. It may help in the recuperative phase of croup if there is a significant amount of mucous production. For dosing, follow the package labeling accurately.
- Valerian root is a mild herbal sedative that may offer some help in easing a child with a significant cough. Valerian root may be most useful at bedtime. For dosing, follow the package labeling accurately.

HOMEOPATHIC REMEDIES (For quick reference please refer to the "Homeopathic Remedies List" on page 32 and the inside cover.)

- A homeopathic remedy designed to support the defense systems in viral infections may be useful. It can be taken 3 to 6 times daily when the virus is active (for example, fever, lethargy, etc.). (General Support 1)
- A homeopathic remedy designed to decrease inflammation and fever from infections may help prevent deterioration and improve the recovery time. It can be taken 3 to 6 times daily when the virus is active (for example, fever, lethargy, etc.). (General Support 2)
- A homeopathic remedy designed to reduce the cough reflex and irritation may be helpful in shortening the duration of the cough. It can be given 2 to 3 times per day until the cough subsides or resolves. (Respiratory 8)

BACH FLOWER REMEDIES

- Rescue Remedy™ may be of use if your child has anxiety with episodes of coughing or stridor. You may use 2 drops every 10 minutes to every few hours to calm restlessness as needed.
- A lukewarm bath with 10 drops of Rescue Remedy™ added to the bathwater is often very effective at relieving agitation and stress in general.

NUTRITIONALS AND SUPPLEMENTS
- Vitamin A
- Vitamin C
- Zinc

DIETARY GUIDELINES
- Avoid mucous-forming foods, especially all dairy products and citrus fruits and their juices.
- Warm foods (soup) and beverages (tea) can often provide temporary relief from a cough.

INTEGRATIVE SUPPORTIVE CARE
- Please read the section "Integrated Management of Respiratory Illnesses."

 When to Call Your Health-care Provider

Call immediately if any of the following occur:
- Stridor that does not improve in spite of the above measures.
- Stridor continues at rest, even when your child is not agitated or crying, and you have tried all the above measures.
- Shortness of breath or rapid breathing rate (over 60 breaths per minute in an infant or over 40 breaths per minute in children over the age of 2 years), especially in the absence of fever.
- Labored breathing in which the chest wall muscles pull in with inspiration.
- Increasing agitation and/or lethargy.
- Blueness of lips or fingernails.
- Difficulty in handling oral secretions, with significant drooling, extremely painful cough (especially in the unvaccinated child).
- High fever in a very ill-appearing child.
- NOTE: If your child stops breathing altogether, dial 911 immediately.

Call within a few hours if:
- Crowing (stridor) only when child is very upset or crying.
- Evidence of dehydration is present. See "Dehydration" section.

Other Relevant Sections

Bronchiolitis

Bronchitis

Colds

Cough

Dehydration

Fever

Throat

Integrated Management of Respiratory Illnesses

Prevention

As noted above, the viral causes of croup are easily transmitted through oral and nasal secretions and are passed from hand-to-eye, hand-to-mouth, or hand-to-nose contact. The virus may also be airborne. Careful hand-washing by parent and child will best help prevent viral spread. You must also be vigilant about your own hand-washing. It is very easy to forget to wash after handling your ill child and his secretions.

Instruct your older child to put his hand over his mouth when coughing and sneezing or to cough and sneeze into his sleeve. Avoid other children known to be ill with cold symptoms, especially during croup season. You will often know from friends, neighbors, and daycare settings that the croup season has begun.

If your child is especially prone to croup, start the humidifier at the first sign of a cold. In this way, you may stay ahead of the swelling and avoid stridor altogether.

A child may develop croup symptoms often during the same season because there are so many different viral triggers. Immunity against one virus gives no protection against another.

DEHYDRATION

 Description/Physiology

Dehydration, although not an illness itself, is a symptom that may be part of many illnesses. It is so common in children that we believe an entire section that describes its causes, expected course, and home treatments would be useful. You will note many references to other sections of this handbook for information on specific triggers. We encourage you to read all relevant sections.

The body is made up of a very high percentage of water, two-thirds by weight. Water is essential to life itself and is involved in every function of the body. Proper hydration is one of the cornerstones of a healthy, balanced child. This means that your child's fluid intake and balance must be sufficient to maintain good blood volume, adequate urine output, lubrication of organs and membranes, temperature regulation, toxin removal, and absorption of nutrients.

When any element of your child's fluid balance (homeostasis) is altered, the potential for dehydration exists. For example, massive vomiting or diarrhea may clearly dehydrate a child. On the other hand, fluid refusal may also put your child at risk for dehydration.

Adequate hydration is especially important during times of illness, as you will see in virtually every section of this book. We include a "hydration" section in nearly every chapter under "Home Care."

Good hydration does many things for the ill child. It helps keep mucous thin and allows mucous flow to remove viruses, bacteria, and inflammatory cells out of the body. Hydration helps the lungs rid themselves of trapped pockets of mucous and infection. A moist mouth, eyes, and nose certainly make a child more comfortable. Good hydration allows the kidneys to work at peak capacity to rid the body of waste products and toxins. Hydration protects the gastrointestinal tract from constipation, helps the gastrointestinal tract rid itself of invading infections, and ensures proper absorption of nutrients and elimination of wastes. The list is endless because every organ and every cell of every organ depends vitally on water.

Hydration is especially critical during fever because fever causes water evaporation.

Here are some very general guidelines about fluid requirements in children. These numbers may vary with each child and the general health of your child, but they will serve as a rough guide for you.

AGE	OUNCES OF WATER PER DAY
2 to 5 years old	12 to 18 ounces
5 to 12 years old	18 to 24 ounces
13 and up	32 to 48 ounces

Causes/Epidemiology

There are hundreds of causes of dehydration in children. They can be grouped into three categories:

1. Abnormally low intake of fluids.

2. Abnormal losses of fluids.

3. Both of the above.

First, regarding abnormal intake of fluids, there are several common themes. For most children who are ill, infants and adolescents alike, the illness may cause a disinterest in and refusal of fluids. The child simply does not want to eat or drink. Other causes of decreased fluid intake include stress and emotional problems, injury, big transitions, teething, earache, the flu, constipation, thrush, and disruption of routines such as travel. The presence of mouth ulcers, such as with Coxsackie virus, the sore throat of strep, or other viruses that produce ulcers or canker sores, will inhibit drinking and eating.

In most cases, when a child decreases his drinking, he may still maintain fluid balance fairly well unless there are simultaneous abnormal fluid losses. Children may have a significantly decreased fluid intake for a few days and be fine, as long as urine output is adequate and there are no other signs of dehydration.

It is rare for a child who refuses to drink to do so for long, unless there is some other serious underlying problem. Thus, fluid refusal rarely, by itself, leads to dehydration.

Second, there are dozens of reasons children may suffer significant fluid losses. Although significant fluid loss may occur at any age, infants and babies are most susceptible to dehydration from fluid losses.

Some of the common causes of abnormal or increased fluid losses and, thus, precursors to dehydration, include:

1. Diarrhea: Triggered by viruses, bacteria, parasites, food intolerances, food poisoning, etc. Please see "Diarrhea" section.

2. Vomiting: Triggered by viruses, bacteria, parasites, food intolerances, head injury, food poisoning, migraines, anatomic problems, etc. Please see "Vomiting" section.

3. Fever: Fever itself causes abnormal fluid loss through heated skin via sweating. It also increases a child's respiratory rate and this increases fluid loss through evaporation of water in the breath.

4. Burns: Significant burns, even sunburn, can be a source of fluid loss.

5. Urinary losses: Substantial fluids may be lost through abnormally large urinary losses, such as with diabetes.

Often these symptoms occur together. The combination of less fluid in and more fluid out puts your child at greatest risk for dehydration.

 ## Expected Course

The course of dehydration depends very much on the age of the child, the cause of the dehydration or illness, and the general health of your child. In most cases, poor hydration may accompany the illness, but the child's own defense system is sufficient to prevent advanced dehydration; however, abnormal losses may overwhelm the child's balance and tip the scale in favor of dehydration.

For infants and babies, fluid reserves are limited. If they develop a diarrhea or vomiting illness, dehydration may progress rapidly. In most cases, if a baby or infant has only 2 to 3 vomiting episodes per day and/or only 2 to 3 diarrhea episodes per day, it is unlikely that dehydration will develop. The greater the number of fluid loss episodes per day, the greater the risk for dehydration.

Initially, these babies and infants will be a bit less active than usual. You may notice some decrease in their urine output and slightly darker urine. Sleep may be disrupted. As the illnesses and dehydration progress, your child may become progressively more lethargic; less interested in drinking or eating; develop dry lips, mouth, and tongue; develop a significantly decreased urine output that may now be dark yellow or brown (brick dust color) and have a more ammonia-like smell; and tears may stop. If an infant or baby does not urinate in 8 hours, dehydration may be present. These children may have sunken eyes, a soft spot that is also sunken, and a pale appearance. Their skin may feel more "doughy." These children are significantly dehydrated and require immediate attention from a health-care provider.

In older children, much the same progression toward dehydration may occur, although the pace is usually slower since older children have a larger volume reserve to deplete. Nevertheless, if abnormal losses are enormous, dehydration may still develop rapidly, even in adolescents.

These children will also become more lethargic and pale. Their urine output decreases and urine is darker. If an older child has not urinated in 12 hours, dehydration has begun. They may be constipated, as well. They may also be excessively thirsty and very irritable. Tear production may cease. Their lips, mouth, and tongue can become dry with thick, white oral secretions.

Children with advancing dehydration must be evaluated either in your health-care provider's office or the emergency room. They will assess the severity of the dehydration and make recommendations about further home care. In some instances, an ER referral will be necessary to analyze blood work, which helps determine the severity of the dehydration, provide intravenous (IV) fluids for hydration, and in some cases, hospitalization for full hydration and observation.

 ## Contagiousness/Immunity

Dehydration is itself not contagious. Viral, bacterial, and parasitic infections that cause diarrhea are all contagious, however.

Your child may return to school or daycare primarily when he is feeling better, the dehydration has been reversed, and the causative agent has been eliminated. The exact point when a child is no longer contagious is difficult to pinpoint. See appropriate sections for causes.

Most of the triggers for dehydration do not confer immunity to your child. Thus, your child may continue to acquire viral infections, even the same ones, year after year.

 ## Home Care

The goals of home care are to relieve discomfort, assess the severity of the overall illness and the degree of dehydration, restore good hydration, and watch carefully for worsening dehydration. Extra parental vigilance is required in infants and babies. We encourage you to review other appropriate sections in this book carefully for guidelines specific to the underlying causes, such as diarrhea, head injury, or vomiting.

We recommend that you read through this entire "Home Care" section first to be sure that you have the proper home approach mapped out for your child's unique situation.

No one cannot anticipate every child's unique situation; that's why your careful observations are essential to seeing this illness through. What follows are general principles to guide you through home treatment and to decisions to seek medical care.

When your child is at risk for dehydration, please begin a log to track the following:

1. Amount and type of fluid drunk in 24 hours.

2. Number and estimated volume of stools/24 hours.

3. Number and estimated amount of vomiting episodes/24 hours.

4. Frequency of urine output (note color, smell). When there is diarrhea at the same time, urine output may be detected by placing a cotton ball over the urethra.

5. Other associated symptoms: fever, abdominal pain, irritability.

6. Presence or absence of tears.

7. Mouth moisture and appearance. (Is it moist and shiny or dry, sticky and having a dull appearance?)

Keep this log as long as your child is ill. It will help you determine whether your child is stable, worsening, or getting better.

There are several principles that apply when trying to halt or reverse dehydration:

1. Determine the cause and treat it, or eliminate it if possible.
   For example, if the cause is food intolerance, eliminate that food.
   If it is a parasite such as giardia, identify it and get treatment for it.

2. Proceed slowly and cautiously with rehydration. Efforts to quickly rehydrate a child using unlimited fluids may cause more diarrhea or vomiting. Try small sips of 1 to 2 teaspoons every 10 to 15 minutes, gradually increasing the volume as is tolerated by your child.

3. In general, dehydrated children do best with clear liquids (which contain small amounts of salts and sugars such as Pedialyte® or ¹/₂ strength Gatorade®) and the avoidance of milk or milk products. (Note: Apple juice may prolong diarrhea.)

4. Avoid red fluids for rehydration as they may look like blood if vomited or stooled.

5. Treat a fever if it is present. Reducing the fever and the aches that often accompany fever may improve a child's interest in drinking and help reverse lethargy and irritability.

6. TLC and patience are vital. Your reassuring touch and nurturing manner will calm your child during this difficult time.

7. Keep the head of your child's bed or crib elevated.

8. Keep the room cool, quiet, and comfortable, and reduce home commotion when possible.

9. Avoid out-of-the-home activity until your child is on the mend.

10. Remember, when your child has ongoing fluid losses (from diarrhea, fever, etc.), he will need his maintenance fluid intake plus replacement of lost fluids.

Depending on the primary symptom or symptoms that have triggered the dehydration, we refer you to:

Diarrhea   See "Diarrhea" section.
Vomiting   See "Vomiting" section.

 ## Integrated Therapies

Note: All of the integrated therapies are directed at providing comfort—for specific interventions refer to the appropriate section, for example, "Vomiting."

(Please refer to the section on "Administering Integrated Treatments" on page 19 for guidance on using any of the therapies that follow.)

AROMATHERAPY

- An aromatherapy bath or massage with the essential oil of lavender can soothe and relax your child's anxiety and restlessness. Add 2 to 5 drops of oil to a warm bath and allow your child to soak for a comfortable period of time.

BACH FLOWER REMEDIES

- Rescue Remedy™ may be of use if your child is uncomfortable from the illness, stress, or anxiety. You may use 2 drops every 10 minutes to every few hours to calm restlessness as needed.
- Ten drops of Rescue Remedy™ added to a lukewarm bath is often very effective at relieving many of the symptoms.

 ## When to Call Your Health-care Provider

Call immediately if your infant or child:
- Becomes so lethargic that he cannot be easily aroused.
- Develops a fever above 105 degrees.
- Develops a stiff neck or is very uncomfortable when moved.
- Is less than 1 year old and has not urinated in more than 8 hours.
- Is older than 1 year and has not urinated in more than 12 hours.
- Has more than 1 stool per hour for 4 consecutive hours.
- Vomits more than twice per hour for 4 consecutive hours.
- Has not made tears in more than 24 hours.
- Vomits blood or has a bloody stool.

DEHYDRATION

Call within 24 hours if:
- Your child is not improving.
- Your child continues to spike fevers in the 104-degree range.
- There is increasing irritability.
- There are still 6 to 8 or more vomiting episodes per day.
- There are still 6 to 8 or more diarrhea episodes per day.

Other Relevant Sections

Colic and The Fussy Baby

Diarrhea

Fever

First Aid—Burns

Head Injury

Influenza

Teething

Urinary Tract Infection

Vomiting

Prevention

Prevention of dehydration depends on the age of the child, the severity and rapid progression of the triggering illness, and the child's immune defenses.

It is always wise to keep your healthy child away from any child known to have an illness that produces loss of body fluids, such as diarrhea or vomiting. For your own ill child, your careful hand-washing will reduce the risk of spread of the virus or bacteria from the ill child to another child or adult via your contaminated hands. Do not share utensils, towels, toys, cups, or books. Encourage your children to wash their hands frequently.

Always keep on hand the appropriate rehydration fluids for your child (under 6 months, plain Pedialyte®; 7 to 24 months, flavored Pedialyte®; and 12 months and older, Gatorade® for you to dilute).

Prevention of dehydration may be successful when rapid identification of risk factors occurs and treatment is instituted immediately.

Description/Physiology

Children in diapers often suffer from diaper rash. Diaper rash may vary from mild to severe, depending on its underlying cause, skin sensitivity, and the frequency of diaper changes. The skin can be red and irritated, dry and peeling, and somewhat tender. The rash may be small spots widely scattered or large patchy areas. Most children will outgrow this tendency by 1 year of age, although sporadic bouts may occur until a child is out of diapers altogether.

 Causes/Epidemiology

The most common trigger of diaper rash is an inflammatory reaction of the skin from contact with the caustic acids and enzymes in urine and/or stool. These acids and enzymes are excreted in the urine and stool in small amounts in the normal child; however, there is increased acid production during an illness or stress (for example, teething, colds, or diarrhea).

Other triggers of contact diaper rash may include disposable diapers themselves, tight plastic pants, commercial diaper wipes, and certain soaps. In some cases, disposable diapers appear to cause diaper rash less frequently than cloth diapers.

Another common cause of diaper rash is yeast. Yeasts live naturally on the skin in relatively low concentrations, controlled by the body's natural immune system. Yeast colonies multiply rapidly in the moist environment of the diaper during an illness or body imbalance. Yeasts have a predilection for inflamed tissue, as well.

Antibiotics also make the skin vulnerable to diaper rash. This may be true even when a breast-feeding mother is taking antibiotics (as small amounts of the antibiotics are passed into breast milk), as well as when the child takes oral antibiotics for a bacterial infection.

 Expected Course

Once the diaper rash has begun, it may progress at either a slow or rapid pace. The irritation may be aggressive enough to cause an erosion of the epidermis (the outer layer of the skin), leaving an open sore which is very tender and may even bleed. Yeast infections appear as a worsening rash of fiery redness, a spreading red border, and/or as smaller "satellite" red pimples/blisters. Nearly all diaper rashes that persist for more than 3 to 4 days have a component of yeast present.

141

DIAPER RASH

In boys, the diaper rash (especially yeast) may be present on the scrotum, shaft, and foreskin of the penis. The scrotum and skin folds can crack and bleed. Treatment in these locations is the same as diaper area skin. In little girls, the labia along with the diaper area may be involved. The labia may be a red color and slightly swollen.

 ## Contagiousness/Immunity

A diaper rash is rarely contagious. Chemical irritation and contact diaper rashes are not contagious at all. Even diaper rashes caused by yeast infections are essentially not contagious. Nevertheless, it is always best to wash your hands carefully after each diaper changing. It is possible to spread the yeast from your hands to the moist diaper area of another child in rare circumstances.

A child does not develop immunity to a contact or yeast diaper rash. Thus, a child susceptible to diaper rashes may develop one often during the first 2 or 3 years of life.

 ## Home Care

The main goal of treatment is to reduce exposure of the skin to the burning acids and enzymes in urine and stool, or other irritants, as well as to provide comfort for your child. This reduced exposure may lessen or even halt ongoing damage to the skin, giving the body's natural healing process time to complete its repair. We ask you to read through the entire "Home Care" section first to determine which of our recommendations make the most sense for your child's current situation.

1. Check your child's diaper at least every 30 to 60 minutes and change any dirty or wet diapers immediately. Even more frequent checks may be necessary if your child has several bouts of diarrhea.

2. With all diaper changes, gently clean all visible stool or urine from the skin with a wet washcloth or diaper wipe. Then, soak the baby's bottom in a basin of clear, warm water for 1 to 2 minutes. This ensures that the invisible film of acid, which is left on the skin after wiping, is removed. You can also rinse your baby's bottom under warm water for 30 to 60 seconds. One other option is to rinse the diaper area with a spray bottle with warm water and then pat dry.

3. Avoid the use of soaps unless absolutely necessary. They may cause discomfort and further irritate damaged skin. If you must use soap for BM removal, use a mild soap like Ivory®.

142

4. Gently blot the skin dry (up and down motion) or allow it to air-dry. You may even use a blow-dryer, aimed from a foot or more distance, on "cool" setting to dry the area.

5. If you suspect a secondary yeast infection, apply Lotrimin® cream (an over-the-counter, anti-yeast cream) first to the rash, and then place your healing cream layer on top of the Lotrimin®. We recommend use of these agents for any diaper rash lasting more than 3 days. This should be done with every diaper change until the rash clears and then for 2 extra days.

6. Apply your favorite "healing" cream, which can be done along with the Lotrimin® cream (above). Popular creams are:

   A. Weleda Baby Calendula Cream® (available at health food stores).

   B. Any cream that contains aloe vera as an ingredient.

7. If the inflammation persists, a low potency steroid cream such as Cortaid®, which is $1/2$% hydrocortisone, can be used twice per day for up to one week.

8. If possible, make time each day for your child to go diaper-free for a time to allow the air to help heal the skin. Best times for open air exposure are after BMs and during naps.

9. When you are ready to re-diaper, you may wish to use barrier creams such as Desitin®, A + D® Original Ointment, or Vaseline® jelly. [NOTE: This should only be done after diaper changes in which you performed Step 2 above.]

10. Good hydration by drinking extra water helps keep urine and stool acids less concentrated and less caustic.

11. If you are breast-feeding your infant, see if there are any allergenic foods in your diet that might be triggering this rash. Some common offenders include dairy products, wheat, nuts, and citrus.

12. If your child develops a diaper rash when new, solid foods are introduced, consider avoiding that specific food until your child is a bit older, and then introduce it again as the only new food for 5 or so days and see if there is a similar reaction.

13. If you are using disposable diapers, consider changing to another brand (especially perfume-free) or a short course of cloth diapers, loosely pinned to allow better air exposure.

14. Commercial diaper wipes are convenient, but their chemical elements may be irritating. Thus, we prefer that you use a soft washcloth and the dip-in-water method for gentler cleansing.

15. If you use disposable diapers, you may poke a number of holes in them to improve air exposure and circulation.

16. An antacid, such as Mylanta® or Maalox®, dabbed on the diaper area may provide another protective barrier.

17. An antibiotic ointment such as Neosporin® may be applied to open sores or cracks of skin to prevent secondary infection.

 ## Integrated Therapies

(Please refer to the section on "Administering Integrated Treatments" on page 19 for guidance on using any of the therapies that follow.)

HERBAL REMEDIES (For quick reference please refer to the "Herbal Remedies List" on page 31 and the inside cover.)

- Calendula extract in a salve or cream base can be applied to the skin directly using the "healing cream" discussion above in "Home Care" section.
- Tea tree oil, for topical use only, has a natural antibiotic and antifungal effect. It can be used to treat diaper rash that has become infected. If the skin appears to become infected, make your own skin wash of tea tree oil by adding 2 to 3 drops of therapeutic grade tea tree oil in 4 ounces of purified water and mix well. This can be gently dabbed onto the diaper area or sprayed on with a spritzer bottle.
- Valerian root is a mild herbal sedative that may offer some help in easing a child with significant restlessness. Valerian root may be most useful at bedtime. For dosing, follow the package labeling accurately.

HOMEOPATHIC REMEDIES (For quick reference please refer to the "Homeopathic Remedies List" on page 32 and the inside cover.)

- A homeopathic cream designed to soothe inflamed or irritated skin may be useful. It can be applied directly to the infected area 3 times a day. (Skin 1)

NUTRITIONALS AND SUPPLEMENTS
- Probiotics

DIETARY GUIDELINES
- Avoid foods that seem to make your child's stools more runny or caustic smelling, such as juices, sugar, etc.

When to Call Your Health-care Provider

Call within 24 hours if:
- The rash does not improve in 3 to 4 days with the above measures.
- The rash spreads rapidly beyond the diaper area.
- The rash develops large open sores, yellow crusting, or bleeding.
- The rash causes enough pain to interfere with sleeping.

Other Relevant Sections

Impetigo

Thrush

Prevention

Although some children are certainly more susceptible than others to diaper rashes, prevention is the key.

We recommend all of the steps outlined above. Anti-yeast medications need not be used preventively. Frequent checks of the diaper for stool and urination, dipping the bottom in water to remove excess urine and stools, patting dry, and placement of a barrier cream are essential to protect this moist area from inflammation and invasion by yeast. Be sure to clean deeper skin folds carefully as they often trap moisture, yeast, urine, and stool.

Cornstarch is not generally recommended. In addition, baby powder is also not recommended. Baby powder can be breathed into the lungs if used several times per day, and the powder particles may cause a chronic cough and even a chemical pneumonia.

Keeping your child's bottom exposed to dry air is helpful. Avoid airtight plastic pants.

The use of a mild detergent soap when washing cloth diapers is recommended.

DIARRHEA

 ## Description/Physiology

Diarrhea is one of the most common and often disconcerting symptoms of childhood. It has many diverse causes. Generally, a diagnosis can be made that pinpoints the cause of diarrhea, and this diagnosis will result in specific recommendations for a direct solution to the problem.

Diarrhea refers to both an increase in the frequency of stools and the water content of the stool. Diarrhea stools may be completely "water loss" or have only a very small amount of texture. These watery stools may be foul-smelling, green or yellow, occasionally bloody, painful to pass, pus- or mucous-streaked, and sometimes explosive.

Diarrhea may be accompanied by increased gas production, a gurgling stomach, abdominal pain, vomiting, and fever. In some cases, diarrhea may be the only symptom present. Other times, all the above symptoms may occur with diarrhea. A diarrhea stool may temporarily relieve the abdominal pain present.

Diarrhea may be the result of poor absorption of food or liquids or the abnormal secretion of stomach and intestinal fluids in response to an infectious or allergic trigger. In addition, there can be poor absorption of the bile acids responsible for absorption of intestinal contents, and these bile acids are further irritants that cause abnormal water loss into the stool.

In breast-fed babies, stools are often very loose, yellow, and contain only a seedy texture. There is often a considerable ring of water around the seedy stool. The stool may be green or yellow. Some breast-fed babies will poop with every feeding. Thus, a baby may have 10 to 12 loose stools per day. This is not diarrhea, but in fact normal breast milk stools.

True diarrhea in a breast-fed infant may sometimes present with blood in the stool, a foul odor, mucous or pus, and/or a dramatic increase in the average number of stools for your infant.

In older children, stool incontinence or watery leakage of stool may occur. Older children can readily give a more accurate account of symptoms to help us reach a diagnosis more quickly.

Diarrhea has a protective function in that it may rid the body of the causative agent—virus or bacteria—naturally. Thus, you must be careful not to rush in with treatment that is too aggressive, until the body has had a chance to do its own repair and healing. This is a fine line, especially in small infants.

Causes/Epidemiology

Milder forms of diarrhea (for example, less than 4 to 5 stools per day) may be a symptom of other health problems, such as colds, teething, etc. Such forms of diarrhea require little or no intervention, as they will generally resolve when the underlying illness goes away with the help of your child's own immune system.

Infectious causes (viruses, bacteria) can be acquired from other children or adults or from water or food contaminated by the agent. The most worrisome forms of diarrhea are usually associated with infections of the intestinal tract.

The vast majority of these infections are viral and are self-resolving. The most common diarrhea viruses are the enteroviruses and the rotavirus. There are, however, dozens of other viral causes of diarrhea. Viral causes of diarrhea occur throughout the year, especially in the summer months. The incubation period for viral diarrhea is usually 2 to 4 days following exposure.

In some instances, diarrhea can be bacterial. These children are generally more toxic in appearance, with fever, bloody stools, and more rapid progression to dehydration. Some bacterial agents include Salmonella, Shigella, and E. Coli.

Another common infectious agent, especially in daycare centers and in the mountains, is giardia. Giardia is a protozoan, an organism that is different from a virus or bacteria. It can cause a long-standing illness with mild, chronic symptoms or a significant illness with intense abdominal pain, significant gassiness, bloody diarrhea, and fever.

Food poisoning may produce very rapid diarrhea in a toxic child who may also have significant abdominal pain and vomiting. Oftentimes, other family members or playmates will be similarly affected and a food source for the poisoning may be traced.

Food allergies or intolerance may also present with diarrhea, including reactions or intolerance to milk and other dairy products. This is especially true in young infants fed cow's milk formulas. It has even been seen in breast-fed babies whose mothers eat dairy products. There may be streaks of blood present in the stool with this "cow's milk colitis."

Some medications can cause diarrhea as a side effect. Antibiotics are the classic trouble-makers. Many antibiotics may also cause abdominal pain, diarrhea, bloating, and even vomiting, due to the direct effect of the antibiotic as well as the change in normal "friendly" intestinal bacteria needed for proper digestion.

Some toddlers have a non-specific form of diarrhea, called "toddler's diarrhea." There is no single obvious cause here, but excessive juice intake may be one possibility. It may also be caused by the high frequency of eating and drinking so common to this age group. Typically, these toddlers have 3 to 4 "soupy" stools per day. There is no problem with the child's growth and essentially no other symptoms present. This form of diarrhea usually resolves by 3 to 4 years of age.

In addition, some children may have starvation stools. Starvation stools occur when a parent feeds a child only clear liquids and no solids for so long that the diet has no bulk to make a formed stool. This usually happens in response to treating a viral-induced diarrhea with prolonged use of clear liquids.

In other instances, over-hydration stools may develop. In this case parents give liquids in excess of the absorptive ability of the intestine, which causes "spilling over" of liquid into a loose stool. This is also frequently a response to overuse of clear liquids when treating viral diarrhea.

Finally, there are many other rare causes of diarrhea, including irritable bowel syndrome, inflammatory bowel disease, or cystic fibrosis.

 ## Expected Course

The course of diarrhea depends on many factors: the cause of the diarrhea, the age of the child, previous foods and medications tried, the general vitality of the child, other concurring problems (such as other acute or chronic illness), and the frequency of stooling.

Most diarrheal illnesses are self-limited, last only 3 to 5 days, and resolve with little or no intervention. They may require only a short period of change of diet. Simple adjustments in formula or milk intake may be all that is necessary.

In more severe instances, anti-diarrheal medications, and even more aggressive therapies such as IV hydration and hospitalization may be needed. These children are considerably more toxic, exhibiting advanced symptoms of dehydration, lethargy, and discomfort.

Dehydration is the key outcome to avoid. Regardless of the cause, dehydration is the most serious result of diarrhea. See "Dehydration" section.

 ## Contagiousness/Immunity

Medication-induced and allergy-triggered diarrheas are not contagious.

Infectious causes of diarrhea, both viral and bacterial, are very definitely contagious to adults and children. They are passed from hand to mouth through fingers contaminated with the infectious agent. They can also be passed from mouth to mouth, that is, by sharing cans of soda, etc. They are generally not airborne.

The most common scenario is a parent or caregiver who changes a diarrhea-laden diaper, is not aware or mindful of the virus or bacteria present on his hands, and then spreads the infectious agent directly to another child's digestive tract (mouth) or his own. Unwashed hands spread the infection easily and rapidly.

A child does not generally develop immunity to the infectious causes of diarrhea. For example, a child with rotavirus can acquire rotavirus every diarrhea season. The same is also true of bacterial causes.

 ## Home Care

The goals in treatment are to provide general suggestions for the prevention of dehydration and the relief of discomfort. Our treatment guidelines should not be taken as a strict recipe, but rather as a general approach for care, with appropriate adjustments made by you, based on your best judgment of your own child.

Observe your child carefully. If he is generally comfortable, not dehydrated, and active between bouts of diarrhea, the body is doing its part to fight off the infection. If, however, your child is progressively more lethargic, inactive, uncomfortable, has a very high fever (above 104 degrees), and exhibits signs of dehydration, there is now cause for greater alarm.

When diarrhea and vomiting are present together, the treatment of vomiting is the top priority. See "Vomiting" section.

We ask you to read through the entire "Home Care" section to select the recommendations that make the most sense for your child's current situation.

Dietary Management

1. Infants 2 to 6 months:

   It is important to record the number of stools your infant produces. Also, make notes of other accompanying symptoms, including vomiting, number of urinations, and fever.

   If there are more than 4 to 5 stools/24 hours:

   A. Discontinue formula for 12 to 36 hours. If you are breast-feeding, you may continue to nurse as long as the "When to Call" criteria listed below are not met; however, continuing to breast-feed may mean slower improvement.

   B. Try Pedialyte® for 12 to 36 hours or until the diarrhea begins to improve. Ideally, you should give 18 to 32 ounces per 24-hour period. Monitor urine output to assure at least one urination approximately every 6 hours.

C. Although your baby may appear hungry all the time or the clear liquids may not seem to satisfy him, try to limit the overall number of feedings to 4 to 5 total feedings per day. Constant "grazing" stimulates the stomach "reflex" that produces more frequent stools. If there is no vomiting present, the feeding size can be anywhere from 4 to 8 ounces/feeding.

D. An infant with diarrhea needs a fluid intake equivalent to normal volume per day plus a replacement volume of 2 to 4 ounces for each liquid stool.

E. Once the diarrhea is under control, you may reintroduce full strength breast milk or formula in a diluted form:

(1) For formula-fed babies, we recommend restarting formula with a soy-based formula, for example, Isomil DF®, at one-third the normal strength (by diluting with extra water) and advance to full strength over a period of 3 to 7 days as dictated by improvement. Increasing the concentration of the formula should be slow and based on whether the increased concentration triggers a return of more diarrhea. For those infants originally on a cow's milk formula (for example: Similac®), you may safely switch back from this temporary soy formula after about 2 weeks on the soy or roughly 3 or 4 days after the diarrhea stops.

(2) For breast-fed infants, we recommend reintroducing breast milk with a decreased number of minutes of nursing and supplement each feeding with Pedialyte®. The Pedialyte® supplement should be weaned over a period of 3 to 4 days while simultaneously increasing the minutes of nursing back to normal. If you are able to pump your breasts and your infant takes a bottle, you may increase the concentration of the breast milk in the same way as formula.

2. Infants 6 to 12 months:

Again, for infants with more than 7 to 8 diarrhea stools per 24 hours:

A. Discontinue milk, formula, and all milk products as well as solid foods. For breast-fed infants, the above recommendations for the 2- to 6-month-old infant may be followed.

B. Give only clear liquids for 12 to 48 hours, depending on the severity of the diarrhea and its response to treatment. Ideally, you should give 24 to 32 ounces of clear liquid per day. The following is a list of clear liquids, and they should all be served at room temperature.

• Pedialyte® (full strength).

- Gatorade® (diluted with water to 1/2 strength).
- Herbal teas.

NOTE: Don't use a red liquid, as it may look like blood in the stool.

C. In 12 to 48 hours, when the diarrhea has improved or is at least stable, begin feeding your child simple, solid foods, especially those solids that are known to be easy to digest and absorb, such as:

- bananas
- applesauce
- rice cereal
- rice
- mashed potatoes
- saltines and dry toast
- cooked carrots
- starchy foods

D. Once these solids are well tolerated, restart cow's milk formula and other milk products. In the older infant, you do not need to use soy products.

E. Administering "probiotics" has been shown to significantly shorten the course and severity of diarrhea (please refer to the "Administering Integrated Treatments" section for guidelines on giving "probiotics" to your child).

3. Children over 1 year:

A. Stop all dairy products for 5 to 7 days and provide liquids from the above list. The ideal amount is 24 to 32 ounces per day.

B. Other acceptable solid foods: the constipating foods listed above; grains (for example, noodles, breads, crackers, and cereals without milk); cooked vegetables; and soft or cooked fruits. Heavy foods such as meat, poultry, and fried foods should be avoided.

C. Administering "probiotics" has been shown to significantly shorten the course and severity of diarrhea (please refer to the "Administering Integrated Treatments" section for guidelines on giving "probiotics" to your child).

D. Over-the-counter medications such as Imodium® AD, Donagel®, and Kaopectate® are of variable effectiveness. Use these medications cautiously and never when there is bloody diarrhea.

DIARRHEA

If the diarrhea persists despite dietary changes described above, you may use Imodium® AD as directed below. Please keep in mind that one dose may be enough to help improve your child's diarrhea. If your child shows no improvement and goes on to have several more loose stools, you may repeat the dose of Imodium® AD. Try to wait 3 to 4 hours between doses and do not give more than 3 doses in a 24-hour period.

Dosages for Imodium® AD

6 - 12 months	$^1/_4$ - $^1/_2$ tsp.
1 - 2 years	$^1/_2$ - $^3/_4$ tsp.
2 - 6 years	1 - 2 tsp.

If your infant or child is not dehydrated, try a period of "bowel rest." In other words, a period of a few hours with no fluids or solids may allow healing time and some improvement of inflammation and the number of stools. This is best accomplished with a long stretch of nighttime sleep or during long naps. The mere act of eating or drinking can trigger the "reflex" that produces a stool.

Pain Relief:

1. Cramping, abdominal pain frequently accompanies diarrhea. If the pain is mostly relieved with a bowel movement, no specific therapy is required. If the abdominal pain persists throughout the illness, without significant relief after bowel movements, you may try either a warm water bottle or a beanbag placed gently on your child's abdomen. Sometimes lying on the side will help.

2. If excess gassiness is present, a trial period of Mylicon® Drops may help to relieve the discomfort from gas and distention.

3. If the pain is more significant or persistent you may try giving Imodium® AD as directed above.

4. If these measures do not help or the pain is intolerable, your child should be seen.

Miscellaneous

1. Diaper rashes are a common side effect of diarrhea in infants and toddlers. See "Diaper Rash" section in this handbook.

2. Antibiotics are rarely used and then only when a specific bacterial source is present. In general, antibiotics will worsen diarrheal illnesses.

Integrated Therapies

(Please refer to the section on "Administering Integrated Treatments" on page 19 for guidance on using any of the therapies that follow.)

AROMATHERAPY

- An aromatherapy bath or massage with the essential oil lavender can soothe and relax your child's anxiety and restlessness. Add 2 to 5 drops of oil to a warm bath and allow your child to soak for a comfortable period of time.

HERBAL REMEDIES (For quick reference please refer to the "Herbal Remedies List" on page 31 and the inside cover.)

- Ginger is a valuable herb that may help in quieting down an "upset stomach," decrease abdominal cramping, and slow down diarrhea. It may be used in the acute phase as well as when the diarrhea is resolving. For dosing, follow the package labeling accurately.
- Mint can also soothe an upset stomach. Mint teas, lightly sweetened, have the added benefit of being an excellent way to get fluids into your child. Mint tinctures are also available. For dosing, follow the package labeling accurately.
- Carob powder can have a beneficial effect on diarrhea, and it is safe for children above the age of 6 months. Carob has a taste similar to chocolate and may be added to soft foods such as applesauce. It can be purchased at any natural food store and many grocery stores. You may give 1/2 to 1 tsp. up to 3 times per day.

HOMEOPATHIC REMEDIES (For quick reference please refer to the "Homeopathic Remedies List" on page 32 and the inside cover.)

- A homeopathic remedy designed to reduce bowel irritation may help decrease the frequency of diarrhea stools. It can be given once with every bowel movement up to 10 times per day until the diarrhea has resolved. (Digestive 3)
- A homeopathic remedy designed to decrease inflammation and fever from infections may help prevent deterioration and improve recovery time. It can be taken 3 to 6 times daily when the virus is active (for example, fever, lethargy, etc.). (General Support 2)
- A homeopathic remedy designed to have a soothing effect on abdominal cramping may be useful. It can be given 3 to 4 times per day as needed for relief of cramping until the diarrhea is relieved. (Pain 1)

BACH FLOWER REMEDIES

- A lukewarm bath with 10 drops of Rescue Remedy™ added to the bathwater is often very effective at relieving agitation and stress in general.

NUTRITIONALS AND SUPPLEMENTS

- Probiotics

DIETARY GUIDELINES

- The most important aspect of dietary management of diarrhea is preventing dehydration through careful fluid management. Please read and follow the guidelines in the "Home Care" section above.
- Encourage foods (age appropriate) that are known to be stool-binding, such as applesauce, cooked carrots, bananas, rice, and toasted foods such as crackers and toast.
- Broth from cooked rice can also be used as a clear liquid during the acute phase of the diarrhea. This can be made by cooking 1/2 to 3/4 cup of brown rice in 4 cups of water. After the rice is cooked, strain the water from the rice. Then use the water according to the guidelines above for clear liquids.
- Rice milk (which can be purchased at natural food stores and almost any grocery store) is a good alternative to milk in the recuperating phase of diarrhea and it has the added advantage of the binding quality of rice. Follow the directions above for re-introducing milk.
- Avoid all foods that are known to loosen stools, such as sugar, fruit juices, prunes, and raw fruits.

 When to Call Your Health-care Provider

Call immediately if any of the following occur:
- A large amount of blood is present in the stool.
- Abdominal pain is severe and intolerable or persists longer than several hours; or the pain localizes to a specific area (for example, the right lower side, as in appendicitis).
- Signs of dehydration have developed. See "Dehydration" section.
- Progressive lethargy and difficulty arousing your child occurs.

Call within 24 hours if:
- The frequency of stools is greater than 8 stools in a 24-hour period.

- A small amount of blood or pus is present in the stool.
- Significant vomiting begins.
- Any signs of worsening dehydration develop.
- Diarrhea began shortly after an antibiotic has been started. (Note: Using a "probiotic" during the course of an antibiotic can minimize the gastrointestinal side effects of the antibiotic. Please see the "Administering Alternative Treatments" section.)

Other Relevant Sections

Colic and The Fussy Baby

Dehydration

Diaper Rash

Fever

Influenza

Vomiting

Prevention

Prevention depends on the cause of diarrhea.

For infectious causes, careful hand-washing after any and all contact with a sick child is essential to prevent spread.

We recommend that you keep your child out of daycare or away from babysitters where diarrhea is known to be a problem. Viral triggers are rapidly spread from child to child and from caregiver to child. Teach your child to wash his hands often at school or in settings where there is considerable contact with other children.

Allergy or food sensitivity triggers should be avoided once they have been identified. In a child less than 5 years of age you should limit juice intake to 4 to 6 ounces per day.

EARACHE/EAR INFECTION

 Description/Physiology

Ear infections and earaches (or ear pain) are very common in childhood. Not all children with ear infections have pain, and many children experience earaches but do not have an ear infection. On average, 80 percent of children develop at least one ear infection in the first two years of life. Ear infections occur most often in children between 6 months and 3 years of age. Ear infections are not emergencies, but they do warrant careful attention.

Ear infections are primarily caused by viruses or bacteria. An earache, on the other hand, may have many causes. Both ear infections and earaches are readily treated either with conventional treatments or through a variety of natural remedies as described below.

A brief bit of anatomy might be helpful here. The ear has three parts: external, middle, and inner. The external ear consists of the pinna (what you see) and the opening, which is called the ear canal. The ear canal leads down to the eardrum, beyond which is the middle ear. The middle ear is the site of ear infections and mucous accumulation. The middle ear has a drainage channel, called the eustachian tube, which connects it to the throat. The properly functioning eustachian tube allows the drainage of mucous out of the middle ear space down into the throat, and thus relieves mucous buildup against the eardrum. A functional eustachian tube helps prevent ear infections. Finally, the inner ear is deeper inside the head and houses special structures for balance, hearing, and perception.

In very young children, the angle of the eustachian tube is fairly flat, which means that mucous does not drain out of the middle ear space as easily as it does in the older child and adult, whose eustachian tubes are angled more sharply. Mucous is trapped more easily in infants and small children. When mucous is trapped in the middle ear space, it can become colonized with viruses and bacteria, which then may lead to an ear infection, also called otitis media.

 Causes/Epidemiology

A true ear infection may be either viral or bacterial. Some medical studies have indicated that viruses cause the majority of ear infections, which explains why so many earaches will resolve without treatment. These viruses are introduced into the body through the mouth, nose, or eyes and produce inflammation of the mucous membranes, which in turn produces mucous in the nose and ear passages. As the mucous accumulates, pressure builds in the

156

middle ear space, pushes against the eardrum and middle ear structures, and causes pain, or the earache.

The body's own immune system generally does a good job of handling viral ear infections. Once the inflammation is calmed, mucous production is reduced, and the residual mucous drains away from the middle ear, thus relieving pain symptoms.

Most bacterial ear infections are secondary infections that are first triggered by a virus. The virus produces mucous as described above, but in this instance, bacteria from the throat or nose colonize the mucous in the middle ear space and multiply rapidly. Any triggers that increase mucous volume or thickness (for example, diets, OTC decongestants, dryness) will increase the risk of secondary bacterial infection. The bacteria form pus collections in the middle ear space, create significant pressure there, and produce pain.

It is important to know that not all earaches are caused by an ear infection. In fact, there are many causes of earache besides a true ear infection, including temporary blockage of the eustachian tube by mucous from congestion; sudden changes in altitude; exposure to cold, outdoor temperatures; and referred pain in conjunction with colds, throat infections, or teething. In these latter cases, pain is "referred" from the throat and gums to the ear region, and this referred pain feels like ear pain.

Overproduction of earwax is rarely a sign of an ear infection. Earwax actually performs a protective function by keeping the ear canal free of inflammation and irritant particles. You do not need to vigorously remove earwax except to reach large plugs that may be blocking the ear canal and that are within easy, visible reach.

Allergies may produce mucous in the middle ear space and can cause pain because of congestion.

There can be occasional trauma to the ear itself. A direct blow to the outside of the ear is obvious. Less obvious is an object inserted into the ear canal that can injure the ear canal or even the eardrum itself. There can be significant bleeding and pain. It is best to have your child examined under these circumstances to be sure that no direct damage has occurred to the eardrum.

An earache may be caused by a foreign body stuck in the ear canal. The object may not be visible to the naked eye. This is common in small children.

Earaches after swimming may be due to an infection of the ear canal, or "swimmer's ear." Swimmer's ear is treated with a topical antibiotic drop. See "Swimmer's Ear" section.

Expected Course

Not all earaches are caused by ear infections. The diagnosis of an ear infection might be suspected due to the pain, but it must be confirmed by your health-care provider's examination.

The course of an ear infection depends on what causes it. In most cases, the child develops a cold characterized by a cough, runny nose, red eyes, and fever. After a few days of these relatively minor symptoms, the child may develop an earache. The earache may be mild to very severe, slow to develop, or abrupt in onset. Some ear pain is excruciating and the child can be inconsolable.

Sometimes an ear infection is accompanied by high fever, swollen glands, and occasional rupture of the eardrum with oozing of pus out of the ear canal.

In young children ear pain may present with pulling on the ears, shaking the head, or simply being very cranky. Ear pulling itself, however, is not necessarily a sign of ear pain and can be caused by factors other than an ear infection. For example, a child may simply be playing with his ears, or pulling may provide some relief from teething or a sore throat. Pulling ears may also be present when a child is tired or cranky or as a habit.

The older child can tell you specifically that his ear hurts. He may report a fullness or pressure and even hearing loss.

We often see pinkeye with pus accompany an early ear infection. The draining eye is frequently on the same side as the ear infection. Pinkeye with pus and ear pain warrant evaluation in your health-care provider's office within 24 hours if symptoms persist. See "Conjunctivitis" section.

You should not ignore signs of general worsening—for example, increased lethargy, temperature greater than 105 degrees, or persistent vomiting.

For children with chronic ear infections, the symptoms may be very similar from one episode to another. You will become quite experienced in diagnosing these symptoms as an ear infection; however, even though the symptoms may appear to be exactly the same as with all previous ear infections, an examination of your child is required to make the correct diagnosis before treatment is begun. There are some rare exceptions to this policy that can be discussed with your health-care provider.

Chronic ear infections may require evaluation by an Ear, Nose, and Throat (ENT) doctor. Hearing testing may be recommended. There may be hearing evaluations done at school that your health-care provider should review, if abnormal.

Contagiousness/Immunity

Bacterial ear infections are not contagious—a child cannot transmit his ear infection directly to another child. However, the virus that may have set the whole process in motion is contagious, so one child with an ear infection can certainly spread his viral infection to another child. Whether that newly infected child will then develop an ear infection is difficult to predict.

Having one ear infection provides no protection against others in the future. In fact, the reverse is often true. Ear infections are rarely isolated, and a first one may signal several others to follow.

Recurrent ear infections (approximately 4 or more in a 12-month period) require careful discussion and assessment of options. Depending on the cause of the infections, a number of possibilities exist, ranging from elimination diets, to ear tubes, to homeopathic treatments, to other natural therapies. This requires a conversation and planning discussion with your health-care provider.

 ## Home Care

The initial goal of treatment is to provide pain relief until your health-care provider can examine your child. We ask you to read through the entire "Home Care" section to select which of our recommendations make the most sense for your child's current situation. The most reliable methods of pain relief include:

1. Warm compresses or heating pad applied to the outside of the ear. Sometimes a cold compress will provide even better relief.

2. Distraction—take your child on a ride, go for a walk, or involve him in a game.

3. Ear drops—these are especially useful. You may use Auralgan® ear drops (by prescription only) or warm oil (salad, vegetable, corn, olive) or Willow Garlic Oil® (available at health food stores). To avoid accidentally burning your child, test the temperature of the oil or Auralgan® first on your own skin before placing it in the ear canal. Place 2 to 3 drops in the painful ear (or both ears if painful ear unknown), and place a cotton plug in the ear canal to keep the drops from draining out. This should be repeated as often as every 15 to 20 minutes until pain is relieved and then as often as necessary after that. Warm the oil each time.

   NOTE: These products cannot be used if your child has ear tubes in place. No pain drops should be used when there is pus drainage from the canal until the ear has been examined.

4. Acetaminophen and ibuprofen. See drug "OTC Medications Recommendations and Dosages" section.

5. Elevate the head of the crib or bed, if possible. This will allow drainage of mucous away from the pressured eardrum.

6. Sucking and chewing may help—a pacifier for infants or a lollypop or chewing gum for older children.

7. Antibiotics may be prescribed for a bacterial ear infection after the diagnosis has been established by your health-care provider's examination. Any antibiotic left over from a previous bacterial infection should never be administered.

    Most antibiotics take 48 to 72 hours to produce definite symptom improvement (including fever), although relief may come sooner. You must use the antibiotics for the recommended number of days (5 to 10 depending on the antibiotic), even if all symptoms have disappeared.

    Immediate relief of pain after 1 or 2 doses of an antibiotic or natural remedy is rare. The fever may persist for the first 2 days while your child is being treated with the antibiotic. In fact, there even may be an elevation of the fever in the first 2 days as the body's immune system rallies to clear the infection.

8. Nasal spray with saline or Ocean® Nasal Spray (see "Colds" section), 2 puffs in each nostril 3 times daily, may help mobilize mucous for better drainage.

9. Good hydration always helps thin mucous.

10. Eliminate dairy products in older children to reduce mucous production.

11. Even if your child's ear pain is gone, it is very important that your health-care provider re-check your child's ears a few days after the therapy has been completed to be certain that the infection and fluid are gone.

12. You can bathe your child and get his ears wet. A warm bath can be a soothing therapy.

13. Do not use earplugs to occlude a pus-draining ear canal. Also, be careful not to get bath or pool water in the ear canal if there is pus draining from the canal.

14. We do not recommend antihistamines or decongestants with ear infections as they tend to thicken the mucous and prevent drainage, and

could thus worsen the pressure and pain.

15. Swimming is permitted once the pain has been relieved, but we discourage diving. Do not let your child swim if there has been a perforation of the eardrum. Traveling to the mountains or on an airplane is safe once the pain has significantly resolved.

16. Earwax need not be removed. It is rare that an earwax impaction causes pain.

Integrated Therapies

(Please refer to the section on "Administering Integrated Treatments" on page 19 for guidance on using any of the therapies that follow.)

AROMATHERAPY

- An aromatherapy bath or massage with the essential oils of eucalyptus radiata and/or lavender can soothe and relax your child's anxiety and restlessness as well as his congestion and difficult breathing. Add 2 to 5 drops of oil to a warm bath and allow your child to soak for a comfortable period of time.

- Add 2 drops each of the essential oils of eucalyptus radiata and lavender to 1 to 2 teaspoons of olive oil and rub on your child's chest to soothe a cough or congestion.

HERBAL REMEDIES (For quick reference please refer to the "Herbal Remedies List" on page 31 and the inside cover.)

- Horehound may be very effective in reducing mucous production. It may help in the recuperative phase of an ear infection if there is a significant amount of mucous production. For dosing, follow the package labeling accurately.

- Valerian root is a mild herbal sedative that may offer some help in easing a child with significant restlessness or pain. Valerian root may be most useful at bedtime. For dosing, follow the package labeling accurately.

- Echinacea/astragalus can be used to support the immune system in helping to resolve a viral infection. For dosing, follow the package labeling accurately.

- Willow bark extract may help an earache as a topical pain reliever. Use the directions above for "Ear drops" in the "Home Care" section and follow the package labeling accurately.

EARACHE/EAR INFECTION

HOMEOPATHIC REMEDIES (For quick reference please refer to the "Homeopathic Remedies List" on page 32 and the inside cover.)

- A homeopathic remedy designed to support the defense system in viral infections may be useful. It can be taken 3 to 6 times daily when the virus is active (for example, fever, lethargy, etc.). (General Support 1)
- A homeopathic remedy designed to decrease inflammation and fever from infections may help prevent deterioration and improve the recovery time. It can be taken 3 to 6 times daily when the virus is active (for example, fever, lethargy, etc.). (General Support 2)
- A homeopathic remedy designed to minimize nasal congestion and mucous, especially when associated with respiratory infections, may be useful. It can be taken 2 to 3 times daily while there is nasal congestion. (Respiratory 3)
- A homeopathic remedy designed to relieve inflammation and drain mucous from the middle ear may be helpful. It can be taken 2 to 6 times a day for 7 to 14 days. (Respiratory 9)

BACH FLOWER REMEDIES

- Rescue Remedy™ may be of use if your child is uncomfortable from the illness, stress, or anxiety. You may use 2 drops every 10 minutes to every few hours to calm restlessness as needed.
- A lukewarm bath with 10 drops of Rescue Remedy™ added to the bathwater is often very effective at relieving agitation and stress in general.

NUTRITIONALS AND SUPPLEMENTS

- Vitamin A
- Vitamin C
- Zinc
- EFAs
- Probiotics

DIETARY GUIDELINES

- It is best to avoid all dairy products and citrus fruits because they may increase or thicken respiratory mucous.
- Warm foods such as soups, warm cooked grains (for example, oatmeal), and teas should be given.
- Cold foods, foods high in sugar, and fried foods should be avoided.

INTEGRATIVE SUPPORTIVE CARE

- Please read the section "Integrated Management of Respiratory Illnesses."

When to Call Your Health-care Provider

Call immediately if any of the following occur:
- You have tried all the above measures for 2 or 3 hours and your child continues to cry inconsolably.
- Blood is draining from the ear.
- An earache is accompanied by increasing lethargy or fever of higher than 104 degrees. It is especially important to notify your health-care provider if your child is unimmunized.

Call within 24 hours if:
- The earache is no better in 12 to 24 hours after trying the above measures.
- Your child's symptoms occur on a weekend or a holiday, and you would like your child examined the next day. Use the above measures to support your child's discomfort during the night. Call the next morning so an exam can be arranged by your health-care provider or a convenient "walk-in" facility.
- The ear infection is no better after 72 hours on the prescribed antibiotic or natural treatment. This may represent a possible failure of the therapy to cure the infection.

 ## Other Relevant Sections

Colds

Conjunctivitis (Pinkeye with Pus)

Fever

Swimmer's Ear

Integrated Management of Respiratory Illnesses

 ## Prevention

It can be difficult to prevent ear infections, but certain common-sense principles apply. For example, if your child often develops an ear infection after a cold, avoid contact with children known to be ill. This is especially true in daycare centers, preschools, and health club nurseries. Cold-prevention techniques (especially careful hand-washing by caregivers and child) are very helpful.

We have found that a combination of dietary changes, air filter treatment, vitamin supplements, some herbal remedies, and/or some homeopathic remedies can have a positive preventive effect on children with chronic ear infections.

Keep your child away from cigarette smoke.

Do not give your baby a bottle in the crib. A baby who sucks a bottle while flat in bed can suck milk into the middle ear space, providing a food source for bacterial growth. Avoid propping the bottle.

If food allergies are the trigger, eliminating these foods once they are identified could significantly reduce the frequency of ear infections. A milk allergy is possible. You should consult with your health-care provider before eliminating certain foods.

If your child is a loud snorer or mouth breather, it is possible that the adenoids are enlarged. These structures, when enlarged, create an obstructive breathing pattern, block the natural flow of mucous, and can lead to recurrent infections of ears, sinus, and throat. In this situation, an evaluation by an ENT and possible adenoidectomy could reduce the frequency of ear infections.

The Prevnar Vaccine is now in widespread use as an immunization directed against the pneumococcal bacterium, one of the leading bacterial causes of ear infections. This vaccine has been shown to reduce the incidence of ear infections in a small percentage of its recipients. You may wish to consult with your health-care provider if your child has not had this vaccine.

Description/Physiology

Eczema is a diagnosis that includes a wide spectrum of rash manifestations and other symptoms. Some of the more common diagnostic terms used to describe these rashes are atopic eczema, atopic dermatitis, dermatitis, and dry skin dermatitis. For the purpose of this section we will include all of the variations under the term eczema.

Eczema is a relatively common problem in children, especially in dry climates. It is rarely a serious problem, but it can produce significant discomfort, principally itching, and may be a challenge to treat.

Eczema is characterized by a skin inflammation that can occur anywhere on the body but most commonly is seen at the skin creases of elbows, knees, behind the ears, and wrists. In an infant, eczema may be seen on the forehead, temples, and behind the neck. The inflammation of eczema can be pink to red. The rash may be patchy, round in shape and raised, and is usually dry and scaly. Itching can vary from mild to intense. It can also be raw and weepy if scratched. Weepy drainage is usually clear or a bit yellow.

The rash may also be generalized to include a sizable surface of the body. Itching and agitation and general irritability are additional primary symptoms.

 ## Causes/Epidemiology

There are many different causes that can trigger eczema, and these different triggering events have led to the variety of terms mentioned above. Food allergies, environmental irritants, genetic predisposition, nutritional and dietary factors, and topical irritants may all play a role in any given child.

Common food allergies such as milk, eggs, and peanut butter may contribute to the development of eczema. Susceptible children in dry climates are far more likely to develop eczema than those living in humid climates. Children with eczema and a strong family history of eczema or asthma are also more prone to asthma themselves. Eczema may also occur from direct contact with irritating substances (for example, soaps, some metals, chlorine, dyes, wool, and plants). Drooling can also trigger eczema around the mouth.

Stress may worsen eczema.

Expected Course

The cause of the eczema will determine how, when, and where the rash will present. Many babies develop eczema within the first two months. This may be due to food allergies (cow's milk formula or foods ingested by a breast-feeding mother) or simply a dry climate. It is usually easily managed with treatments suggested below, but it can also evolve beyond the common sites and into a diffuse and significant rash. It may cover a large portion of the baby's body. Patches of redness may coalesce into entire sheets of dry rash.

Itching and general agitation are very common. The greater the surface area involved, the more uncomfortable your child. Occasionally, a child may scratch so intensely as to cause bleeding and even secondary bacterial infections such as impetigo. The scalp and face can be particularly troublesome.

If the triggers for eczema are eliminated, most of the time it will improve dramatically. However, even with proper treatment and routine preventive measures, there may be occasional flare-ups.

Most infants and young children with eczema will outgrow the disease; however in some, it may become a chronic condition and can persist until adolescence. When this happens, the skin thickens and becomes a scaly rash, with yellow and deep-red areas.

In general, your health-care provider can usually manage the disease with office treatments, but on occasion, they may seek the advice of a dermatologist or allergist.

 ## Contagiousness/Immunity

Eczema is not contagious. Children with visible eczema may mistakenly be perceived as having a contagious illness, however. Proactive communication with child-care providers and play-group parents may prevent misunderstanding and anxiety.

 ## Home Care

Early treatment and preventive measures are the keys to avoiding severe eczema. The goals of therapy are to reduce and prevent itching and provide comfort and relief to the agitated child. We ask you to read through the entire "Home Care" section to determine which of our recommendations make the most sense for your child's current symptoms.

These measures include:

1. Bathing and hydrating the skin. Your child with eczema may have a bath every day, but you should not use soap more than once or twice a week. Problem areas (diaper area) may be washed separately as needed in a sponge bath. Fewer soap baths allow the skin to restore and maintain its own natural, lubricating oils. Moisturizing oil, such as sesame or almond oil (if no nut allergies), may be used in the baths of older children.

    Eczematous skin is very sensitive to soaps. So, young infants can be washed without any soap at all. Older children will need a mild soap, such as Dove®, Cetaphil®, or a glycerin-based soap for proper cleansing. Do not allow your child to soak in a soapy tub. Rinse shampoo and all soap thoroughly from the skin at the end of the bath or shower.

2. Lubricating cream. After a 5-minute bath, your child's skin is well-hydrated. This is the best time to trap moisture into the still-damp skin by applying a generous layer of cream to the entire skin surface. Lubricating cream can also be applied 2 or 3 times daily at least or more often if needed. Spraying a fine mist of water onto the skin first, before you apply the cream, will help even more to hydrate the skin.

    We recommend any of the following lubricating creams: Weleda Baby Calendula®, Keri®, Lubriderm®, Nivea®, Nutraderm®, Eucerin®, Kiss My Face®, Cetaphil®, or Aquaphor®. Avoid applying any ointments, petroleum jelly, or vegetable shortening because these agents may block sweat glands, increase itching, and worsen the rash.

3. Itching therapy. At the first sign of any itching, apply moisturizing cream to this area. Keep your child's fingernails cut short. On occasion, it may be necessary to give your child oral Benadryl® to reduce acute itching. See "OTC Medication Recommendations and Dosages" section. These preparations may cause drowsiness, however, so they should be used cautiously. A cool, wet compress can relieve especially intense itching. A room humidifier will help moisten skin and reduce itching.

4. Steroid creams. Steroid cream (for example, one-half percent or 1% hydrocortisone cream or Cortaid®) may be an important treatment for eczema. Apply a thin layer of cream 3 times daily to the rash in the most inflamed skin areas where eczema flares. When the rash quiets down, usually within 1 to 2 days, use Cortaid® at least once daily for 3 to 4 more days until the inflammation has disappeared. After that, use it on any spot that itches and appears particularly red and dry. Steroid creams should not be used for longer than 2 weeks at a time (without the specific direction from a health-

care provider). Cortaid® is available over-the-counter. Cortaid® is best reserved for the reddest areas and is not recommended daily for simply dry skin. Dry skin alone is best treated with lubricants. Minimize the use of steroid creams on the skin of the face and the groin/genital area. Contact your health-care provider for specific advice for treating these areas.

5. Diet. Certain foods can be eliminated from the diet, and this may improve eczema. Common triggers include milk, nuts, shellfish, soy, wheat, eggs, and citrus. In some cases, these allergens will pass into breast milk and may cause eczema in the breast-feeding infant. If you suspect that several food groups will need to be eliminated, contact your health-care provider for nutritional advice.

6. Sunscreen. Eczematous skin is especially prone to sunburn, so be very mindful of the time spent in the direct sunlight. Sunscreen should be applied before any sun exposure.

7. Relaxation. Older children may respond to relaxation techniques.

 ## Integrated Therapies

(Please refer to the section on "Administering Integrated Treatments" on page 19 for guidance on using any of the therapies that follow.)

AROMATHERAPY

- German chamomile applied topically in a carrier oil can be very effective in relieving the symptoms of eczema. It may also be applied as a skin wash.

HERBAL REMEDIES (For quick reference please refer to the "Herbal Remedies List" on page 31 and the inside cover.)

- (NOTE: Because echinacea is an immune stimulant, we do not recommend its use in diseases in which the immune system is overactive, such as asthma or eczema.)

- Calendula extract in a cream base can be applied to the skin directly instead of the hydrocortisone cream discussed above in the "Home Care" section.

- Tea tree oil, for topical use only, has a natural antibiotic and antifungal effect. It can be used to treat or prevent eczema from becoming infected. If the skin appears infected, use the tea tree oil 2 to 3 times a day, or as a preventive it can be used 2 to 3 times a week. A tea tree oil skin wash, gel, or cream is best as the full strength oil is too strong for your child's skin. To make tea tree oil skin wash, add 10 drops of therapeutic grade tea tree oil to 1 ounce of purified water and apply 3 times a day with a cotton pad or from a spray bottle.

- Valerian root is a mild herbal sedative that may offer some help in easing a child with a significant restlessness or itching. Valerian root may be most useful at bedtime. For dosing, follow the package labeling accurately.

HOMEOPATHIC REMEDIES (For quick reference please refer to the "Homeopathic Remedies List" on page 32 and the inside cover.)

- A homeopathic remedy designed to reduce the symptoms of skin irritation and breakdown may promote healthy skin. It can be taken 2 to 3 times daily for up to 3 weeks as long as the rash is improving. (Skin 2)
- A homeopathic cream designed to soothe inflamed or irritated skin may be useful. It can be applied directly to the affected area 3 times a day. (Skin 1)
- A homeopathic remedy designed to decrease inflammation from infections and other irritants may help prevent deterioration and improve the recovery time. It can be taken 3 times daily for up to 3 weeks as long as the rash is improving. (General Support 2)

BACH FLOWER REMEDIES

- Rescue Remedy™ may be of use if your child is uncomfortable from the illness, stress, or anxiety. You may use 2 drops every 10 minutes to every few hours to calm restlessness as needed.
- A lukewarm bath with 10 drops of Rescue Remedy™ added to the bathwater is often very effective at relieving agitation and stress in general.

NUTRITIONALS AND SUPPLEMENTS

- Vitamin A
- Vitamin E
- EFAs (In eczema, "evening primrose oil" may be substituted for flax oil in the same dose.)
- Probiotics

DIETARY GUIDELINES

- Avoid any food your child is allergic to or which you suspect makes his eczema worse.

When to Call Your Health-care Provider

Call within 24 hours if:
- The rash appears to be infected or your child has a fever from the infection.
- The rash becomes raw and bleeding.
- The rash hasn't improved after 7 days of the above treatment.
- The itching interferes with sleep in spite of the above treatment.
- The rash becomes very tender in certain areas.
- Your child with eczema contracts chickenpox.

 ## Other Relevant Sections

Athlete's Foot

Diaper Rash

Hives

Impetigo

 ## Prevention

Daily lubrication, avoidance of certain troublesome foods, and avoidance of skin irritants are very important aspects of eczema prevention. For example, wool fibers and clothes made of other scratchy, rough materials worsen eczema. So, all-cotton clothes should be worn.

Avoid other eczema triggers, such as excessive heat, excessive cold, very dry air (use a humidifier), chlorine, harsh chemicals, and soaps. Don't use bubble bath. Avoidance of specific eczema-worsening foods (milk, wheat, etc.) is important.

Double rinsing of your child's clothes, bedding, and towels in the washer removes residual, irritating laundry soap which can be an irritant. A mild laundry detergent such as Dreft® or allergy-free detergents such as Cheer Free® can help. Avoid the use of scented fabric softeners or dryer sheets.

Description/Physiology

Fever is the single symptom that worries parents most. It is the symptom about which pediatricians field the most questions. We hope this discussion will relieve your fears and sensitively guide your treatment of your feverish child.

Children with fever may be irritable, flushed, a bit sweaty, and restless; they may complain of achiness and pain and have a decreased appetite. Many will also have other symptoms from the underlying illness trigger—diarrhea, cough, runny nose, rash, and vomiting. Over a prolonged period of time, decreased fluid intake and the evaporative losses of fluid from the skin and breathing may cause dehydration.

Fever is the body's natural response to an infection or invading agent. It is much like a self-produced "antiviral" or "antibiotic" in that it helps the body fight the attacking infection. An elevated temperature may naturally destroy the infecting agent directly, and so we view a fever as part of the body's natural defense system. The fever may also increase the immune response and effectiveness—for example, by increasing the activity of white blood cells, which themselves act against the invading infection. So some fever may be good, but the discomfort that it causes may need to be addressed.

There is often confusion about what a true fever is in a child. Here is our approach to fever management. A temperature of less than 100.0 degrees is considered normal in all children. The body's normal temperature range can be 97.5 to 100.0 degrees (rectal or oral) during a 24-hour period. Measuring 98.6 degrees exactly is unlikely. So, at any given time of the day, the core body temperature can vary plus or minus 2 degrees, depending on the level of your child's activity, the amount of clothing worn, and the environmental temperature. Body temperature runs a bit higher in the evening than during the day.

The height of the fever may not necessarily be an indication of the severity of the illness. Children with a mild cold may have a surprisingly high fever. On the other hand, children with more serious illnesses, such as pneumonia, may have only a low-grade fever. Thus, the height of the fever itself can be a bit misleading.

A high fever, in and of itself, is not dangerous. Most fever is handled effectively by the body and a fever stops climbing naturally. Fevers above 106 degrees are extremely rare and are generally associated with external over-heating of a child—for example, a child left in a hot car. Fortunately, children tolerate fever well (certainly better than adults!). Children are more likely to have a higher fever and to have a more rapid rise in fever than adults.

FEVER

There are a number of myths about fevers that can cause great concern on the part of parents and caregivers. The following statements are the known facts about fevers and their impact on children:

- Fevers in and of themselves are not harmful to children.
- Fevers do not cause brain damage.
- Fever seizures are not harmful.
- Without treatment, fevers do not continue to go higher and higher. They tend to "top out" at 105 to 106 degrees.
- Even with treatment, most fevers may not come down exactly to normal body temperature.
- Even if the fever does not come down with treatment, the cause is not always serious.
- Bringing the fever down with acetaminophen or ibuprofen does not "cure" the underlying illness, nor does it make the child non-contagious to others.

The exact degree of the fever is far less important than how your child looks! If your child looks sick, even with a low-grade fever, this is more cause for concern than the child who runs around with a temperature of 104 degrees and no other symptoms!

 ## Causes/Epidemiology

Fevers can be caused by many factors. Viral infections, such as a cold or flu, are probably the most common causes of a fever in children. In addition, bacterial infections, such as ear infections, urinary tract infections, strep and pneumonia, may produce a fever as one of their many symptoms.

Less common causes of fever include an allergic or toxic reaction to a bite or drug, autoimmune disease, sun exposure, dehydration, overexertion, etc. In some cases, we never discover the cause of a fever. A "Fever of Unknown Origin" (FUO) is defined as a fever lasting more than 7 days for which no cause can be determined.

 ## Expected Course

The course of a fever depends on its cause. In viral infections, the fever is present in the range of 100.5 to 105 degrees for an average of 3 to 5 days. There can be wide swings of fever during the day. These fevers will generally respond well to anti-fever medications such as ibuprofen or acetaminophen. In the case of viral influenza, for example, the fever is quite high in the beginning days of the illness and then tends toward lower levels as the infection resolves.

In bacterial infections, fevers vary widely from low grade to higher depending on the severity of the disease. The fever of a bacterial infection can range from 100.5 to 106 degrees. A fever from a bacterial infection may continue and in many cases worsen, until proper antibiotic treatment has begun.

After the fever has been reduced with acetaminophen or ibuprofen, most children will look and feel noticeably better, begin to eat more normally, and increase their activity level. They may sleep better. This "honeymoon" period may be short-lived until the medication "wears off," so your child should be kept at rest. Some children attempt to return to normal activity during this improved phase, only to have a return of fever and lethargy when the medicine wears off.

Some children with high fevers will become delirious or hallucinate. They may see things crawling in their bedroom, not immediately recognize you, and act restless and very agitated. While these symptoms are dramatic and usually frighten parents, they are not dangerous and resolve when the fever is reduced.

We are often asked about "fever seizures" or "febrile seizures," which do occur, though not commonly. Most fever seizures are not related to either the rapid rise in temperature or the height of the fever. Often they occur before you realize that your child is ill. Thus, they are difficult to anticipate.

Fortunately, fever seizures are not a dangerous type of seizure and pose no serious threat to your child. After a first episode of a febrile seizure, parents are encouraged to treat fevers more aggressively, even low-grade ones, at the first signs of an illness. Febrile seizures occur primarily in young children (less than 5 years old); many recur in the same child and are usually outgrown within a few years of their onset. Fever seizures tend to be hereditary.

A common myth, which is frequently asked about, is whether or not high fevers can cause "brain damage." In normal children, brain injury from a high fever does not occur, even at temperatures as high as 106 degrees.

Contagiousness/Immunity

Fever is a usually a symptom of an infection. While the fever itself is not contagious, the underlying infection that is causing the fever is probably contagious. Therefore, you should consider your child contagious when he has a fever unless your health-care provider determines he is not contagious. The usual precautions for disease spread should be observed.

In terms of immunity, whether a child develops immunity to an infection depends on the child and the infectious agent. For example, it is rare to develop chickenpox twice. On the other hand, a child can acquire the same viral agent (such as a cold) every season.

 ## Home Care

When a fever occurs, we ask you to consider several factors. First, assess the overall "look" of your child. Ask yourself a few basic questions: How is my child acting? Is my child eating well? Are there other symptoms present—lethargy, irritability, restlessness, poor sleeping, and complaints of pain? Are other family members ill?

This kind of information will be very useful in assessing the severity of the illness and the fever.

These are the ways that we, as providers, describe a fever:

100° to 101.9°	Low-Grade Fever
102° to 103.9°	Moderate Fever
104° to 106°	High Fever

If you suspect a fever, we recommend that you measure your child's temperature once to document the presence of a true fever. This is because many children "feel warm" to the touch (especially on the head and chest), but their core body temperature may actually be within the normal range. These large areas radiate much body heat and may lead you to suspect a fever. But when the actual temperature is measured, it is often less than 100.5 degrees, and thus is normal. That's why thermometer documentation of a fever is useful at least once. We encourage you to take the temperature infrequently, not several times a day.

A 3-minute rectal temperature (in children less than 5 years), or in the older, more cooperative child, a 3-minute oral temperature measurement, are the most accurate. In younger children and infants, an axillary (under the arm) temperature measurement should be taken for a full 5 minutes. The axillary temperature may be slightly different from an oral or rectal temperature; however, we prefer that you simply report the actual temperature that was measured and where you measured it.

The glass thermometer and the digital electronic thermometer are accurate when used properly. Ear thermometers are also fairly accurate in children 4 months of age and older, but are expensive. Temperature strips for forehead measurement are unreliable, so they are discouraged.

We ask you to read through the entire "Home Care" section first and select which of our recommendations make the most sense for your child's current situation.

1. If your infant is two months of age or younger, has not just received immunizations, and has a fever of 100.5 or higher, call your health-care provider immediately before you do anything else.

2. If your child is older than 2 months of age, has a temperature of greater than 100.0 degrees and seems well otherwise (eating well, alert, and smiling), you need not give medication to lower the temperature right away. By waiting a bit to start anti-fever medication, you allow the fever to do its own natural work to fight the infection. This is the time for careful observation and patience on your part. Premature lowering of a fever with medications may interfere with your child's own immune system response to destroy the germs causing the fever. This approach may confuse and alarm friends and relatives who are accustomed to immediate treatment even for low-grade fevers.

3. If your child is older than 2 months of age, has a fever, and is uncomfortable, you may try the following measures to reduce discomfort:

    A. Give acetaminophen every 4 hours as needed. See "OTC Medication Recommendations and Dosages" section.

    B. You may try ibuprofen. See "OTC Medication Recommendations and Dosages" section. In general, we recommend ibuprofen in children only over 6 months of age because of its anti-fever effect as well as its anti-inflammatory effect. We believe that it is better than acetaminophen at reducing the achy discomfort that accompanies a fever. Both ibuprofen and acetaminophen are analgesics and thus provide relief of the aches associated with fever.

    C. Never use aspirin in place of acetaminophen or ibuprofen.

    D. Increase fluid intake (Pedialyte®, Gatorade®, juice, water, popsicles, etc.). See "Dehydration" section. Fever causes the loss of body fluids through evaporation from the skin and through breathing more rapidly. Thus, children with fevers are more prone to dehydration. Give your child as many liquids as he wants.

    E. Keep clothing to a minimum. Loose, light cotton clothes are best. In babies, a diaper alone will be fine. Keep your child out of a draft. Do not bundle your child up. This is especially true for infants.

If your child is still uncomfortable after the above measures, you may immerse him in a lukewarm bath. The bath water should be the same temperature as a normal bath, because that will still be much cooler than your child's body temperature when he has a fever. Never bathe your child in an alcohol or cool water bath, as this will cause your child to chill and shiver, which can actually cause the temperature to rise. The main purpose of a lukewarm bath is to ease the aches and pains associated with a fever. While it may have the effect of also reducing the body temperature, comfort is really the goal. You may also use a sponge bath, sponging as much of the body and head as possible. Because of the cooling effect of evaporation of the water from the skin, a sponge bath may be more uncomfortable. The bathroom itself should be warm enough to keep your child from shivering, because shivering will actually cause a rise in body temperature.

Dosing Notes

- There may be a significant difference between the dosage of drops and elixir forms of acetaminophen and ibuprofen. Be sure to note which preparation you have and use the dropper or measuring spoon packaged with that specific product. Always consult our "OTC Medication Recommendations and Dosages" section for specific guidelines according to age, weight, and type of medication.
- Avoid using ordinary spoons to measure medications. This way of measuring doses may be inaccurate. For exact dosing, use the pre-packaged measuring syringe/spoon or pick up a dosing syringe at your health-care provider's office or your pharmacy.
- Using acetaminophen or ibuprofen at the same time as other medications (for example, antibiotics, cold medications) is fine, as long as the other medication does not also contain acetaminophen or ibuprofen. Check the package carefully for all ingredients of other medications you administer.
- Do not awaken your child to administer acetaminophen or ibuprofen. Sleep is essential for healing, and if your child is comfortable enough to sleep even with a fever, he should remain asleep. However, check on your child during sleep to be sure that no new symptoms have developed—more labored breathing, color changes, unusual rash, etc. It is reasonable to awaken your child at least once during the night to be sure that he is easily arousable.
- Acetaminophen or ibuprofen may not always reduce your child's temperature to "normal" (98.6 degrees). Remember, our goal is to treat your child's discomfort, not just "the number."
- It takes approximately one hour for both ibuprofen and acetaminophen to lower a fever.

- If your child is vomiting and can't keep any medication down, please try a rectal suppository form of acetaminophen. These are available over-the-counter but are usually stocked behind the pharmacy counter as they require refrigeration. Follow directions as indicated on the label.
- Alternating acetaminophen and ibuprofen probably provides little or no real benefit to reduce fever because both drugs work by similar mechanisms. In some circumstances, however, it may improve pain relief. If you choose to use both medications, caution should be used. Generally, we recommend starting with a first dose of ibuprofen and then 3 hours later a dose of acetaminophen. This is followed in 3 more hours by a dose of ibuprofen and then in 3 more hours by another dose of acetaminophen, and so on. The dose of each medication should be carefully measured and double-checked to avoid confusion. It is a good idea to keep a written log of each dose that you give, to minimize the risk of incorrect dosing or overdosing. The acetaminophen and ibuprofen should be alternated on an every-3-hour basis.

 ## Integrated Therapies

(Please refer to the section on "Administering Integrated Treatments" on page 19 for guidance on using any of the therapies that follow.)

HERBAL REMEDIES (For quick reference please refer to the "Herbal Remedies List" on page 31 and the inside cover.)
- Use remedies that are specific for the underlying illness.
- Valerian root is a mild herbal sedative that may offer some help in easing a child with significant restlessness. Valerian root may be most useful at bedtime. For dosing, follow the package labeling accurately.

HOMEOPATHIC REMEDIES (For quick reference please refer to the "Homeopathic Remedies List" on page 32 and the inside cover.)
- A homeopathic remedy designed to decrease inflammation and fever from infections may help prevent deterioration and improve the recovery time. It can be taken 3 to 6 times daily when the virus is active (for example, fever, lethargy, etc.). (General Support 2)

BACH FLOWER REMEDIES
- Rescue Remedy™ may be of use if your child is uncomfortable from the illness, stress, or anxiety. You may use 2 drops every 10 minutes to every few hours to calm restlessness as needed.

177

• A lukewarm bath with 10 drops of Rescue Remedy™ added to the bathwater is often very effective at relieving agitation and stress in general.

DIETARY GUIDELINES

• It is best to avoid all dairy products and citrus fruits because they may increase or thicken respiratory mucous.
• Warm foods such as soups, warm cooked grains (for example, oatmeal), and teas should be given.
• Cold foods, foods high in sugar, and fried foods should be avoided.

 When to Call Your Health-care Provider

Call immediately if any of the following occur:
• Your child is less than 2 months old and has a fever of greater than 100.0 degrees.
• At any temperature your child is markedly uncomfortable or inconsolable, especially after the use of acetaminophen or ibuprofen.
• Your child appears more ill than can be accounted for by the fever alone. For example, after the temperature is lowered your child is still very lethargic, difficult to arouse, or very uncomfortable.
• Your child's temperature is greater than 105 degrees.
• Your child has a seizure.
• Your child has a very stiff neck or severe headache, refuses to move, cries intensely with movement, and/or is upset when you try to move him.
• Your child has developed symptoms of dehydration. See "Dehydration" section.
• Your child continues to have rapid breathing or an increased work of breathing even after the fever has been lowered.
• Your child is ill-appearing with a fever and has not been immunized.

Call within 24 hours if:
• Fever alone persists more than 3 days without other associated symptoms.
• Fever returns after a 1- to 2-day absence during the same illness.
• Your child spikes a fever 2 to 3 days after starting antibiotics.

- Your child's fever does not disappear after 3 days of antibiotic treatment for a bacterial infection.
- Your child complains of burning with urination. See "Urinary Tract Infection" section.
- Your child complains of an earache. See "Ear Infection" section.

 ## Other Relevant Sections

Colds

Croup

Dehydration

Infectious Mono

Influenza

Urinary Tract Infection

OTC Medication Recommendations and Dosages

Integrated Management of Respiratory Illnesses

 ## Prevention

Prevention depends largely on the cause of the fever. In most cases, there is no need to initially prevent the fever, because in doing so, we may interfere with the body's natural response.

Keep your child away from other adults and children with infections. This is especially true in settings where many children come together, such as daycare centers. Remember to teach and practice good hand-washing.

Prevention of fever is important in children less than 3 years of age who have suffered a previous febrile seizure. Prompt treatment with ibuprofen and/or acetaminophen at the very beginning of an illness that is likely to trigger a fever (colds, diarrhea, croup) is prudent.

FIFTH DISEASE

(Erythema Infectiosum)

 ### Description/Physiology

Fifth disease is a viral illness seen most commonly in children 2 to 8 years of age. It is generally a benign infection that lasts for only a few days and rarely requires treatment. Of historical interest, "fifth disease" got its name when pediatricians attempted to categorize the infectious illnesses of childhood that were associated with a red rash. There were five such illnesses (for example, measles) and they decided to simply name the fifth one "fifth disease."

 ### Causes/Epidemiology

Fifth disease is caused by the Human Parvovirus B19. This virus is quite common and can easily sweep through daycare centers, sporting club nurseries, and preschools.

 ### Expected Course

Fifth disease is characterized by a red rash on both cheeks, often described as a "slapped cheeks" appearance. This rash lasts approximately 1 to 3 days. The red facial rash is usually followed by a pink, "lace-like" rash on the extremities and/or trunk. This rash looks a bit like a "fish net" in appearance. This second rash may fade and then reappear, on and off again for 3 weeks. The rash itself is usually the defining symptom. There may be a low-grade fever or no fever at all. Appetite and sleep are rarely disrupted.

 ### Contagiousness/Immunity

Because it is a viral disease, fifth disease is contagious. It can be transmitted through direct secretion contact from person to person. Adults may transmit the virus to children and vice versa. The disease may go virtually unnoticed in adults or adolescents. Fifth disease is less likely to be transmitted in the air.

A child develops some immunity to fifth disease, but may also acquire it again the next year. Because the disease is mainly contagious during the week before the rash appears, a child who has the rash is no longer considered contagious and can return to school or daycare. It is important to keep these children away from pregnant women.

Pregnant Women Exposed to Fifth Disease. Recent research shows that approximately 10 percent of fetuses infected with fifth disease develop severe anemia. This virus, however, does not cause any other birth defects. Fortunately, the likelihood of this happening in the general population is quite rare. We estimate that only 1 in 20,000 pregnancies are at risk. If you are pregnant in your first trimester and exposed to a child with fifth disease, call your obstetrician. Your obstetrician may draw a sample of your blood for an antibody test to determine whether you have already had the disease and are thus protected from re-infection. If you do not have antibodies against fifth disease, your pregnancy will need to be monitored more closely as directed by your obstetrician.

 ## Home Care

No specific treatment is generally necessary other than general supportive care. The distinctive rash of fifth disease is harmless and causes no symptoms that require treatment. If your child is a bit lethargic from a low-grade fever, you may administer acetaminophen or ibuprofen. See "OTC Medication Recommendations and Dosages" section. As always, rest and good hydration will speed healing.

 ## Integrated Therapies

(Please refer to the section on "Administering Integrated Treatments" on page 19 for guidance on using any of the therapies that follow.)

HERBAL REMEDIES (For quick reference please refer to the "Herbal Remedies List" on page 31 and the inside cover.)

- Aloe vera or calendula applied topically can reduce itching and soothe irritated skin. They are available in gel, lotion, or cream. For dosing, follow the package labeling accurately.
- Valerian root is a mild herbal sedative that may offer some help in easing a child with a significant restlessness. Valerian root may be most useful at bedtime. For dosing, follow the package labeling accurately.

HOMEOPATHIC REMEDIES (For quick reference please refer to the "Homeopathic Remedies List" on page 32 and the inside cover.)

- A homeopathic remedy designed to support the defense system in viral infections may be useful. It can be taken 3 to 6 times daily when the virus is active (for example, fever, lethargy, etc.). (General Support 1)

- A homeopathic remedy designed to decrease inflammation and fever from infections may help prevent deterioration and improve recovery time. It can be taken 3 to 6 times daily when the virus is active (for example, fever, lethargy, etc.). (General Support 2)

BACH FLOWER REMEDIES

- Rescue Remedy™ may be of use if your child is uncomfortable from the illness, stress, or anxiety. You may use 2 drops every 10 minutes to every few hours to calm restlessness as needed.

DIETARY GUIDELINES

- Warm foods such as soups, warm cooked grains (for example, oatmeal), and teas should be given.
- Cold foods, foods high in sugar, and fried foods should be avoided.

INTEGRATIVE SUPPORTIVE CARE

- Please read the section "Integrated Management of Respiratory Illnesses."

 When to Call Your Health-care Provider

Call within 24 hours if:
- Your child develops a fever over 103 degrees.
- The rash changes significantly and becomes more hive-like, purplish, and tender.
- Your child becomes progressively more lethargic or inconsolable.
- Your child complains of a progressive sore throat.
- Your child appears to be developing jaundice, or a more yellow skin tone, or he seems especially pale and more easily fatigued.

 Other Relevant Sections

Fever

Hives

Throat

Integrated Management of Respiratory Illnesses

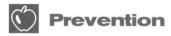 Prevention

Prevention is made difficult by the fact that a child's most contagious period is before the "slapped cheek" rash appears. As always, careful hand-washing by adults after handling an ill child is important.

HAND, FOOT & MOUTH DISEASE

(COXSACKIE VIRUS OR HERPANGINA)

 ### Description/Physiology

Hand, foot, and mouth disease is a common and highly contagious viral infection characterized by small, deep, painful ulcers in the mouth. These mouth ulcers are especially painful on the tongue and the back of the throat. The gums are not usually involved. Hand, foot, and mouth disease occurs primarily in children 6 months to 4 years of age.

There may also be dozens of small blisters or red spots on the palms of the hands and the soles of the feet. In some cases, there may only be a few scattered blisters. Rarely, the blisters can be seen on the buttocks and legs. These blisters initially may be confused with the blisters of chickenpox, but unlike the much wider distribution of the chickenpox rash, they are confined to the palms and soles and mouth.

Occasionally these mouth ulcers occur in the absence of blisters on the palms and soles. This variation, often referred to as "herpangina," is not caused by the "herpes" virus, although coxsackie and herpes viruses are related to each other.

 ### Causes/Epidemiology

Hand, foot, and mouth disease is caused by the Coxsackie A virus. It is not the same virus as the hoof and mouth disease of cattle. Coxsackie season occurs typically in the warmer months of the year.

 ### Expected Course

A child will typically present with fever and general discomfort lasting 3 or 4 days. The mouth ulcers develop about the same time as the fever and resolve within 7 days, but the blisters/rash on the hands and feet can persist up to 10 to 12 days. Children may be very fussy during the first few days. Sleep may be disrupted.

The primary complication we see is dehydration. Dehydration results when children refuse to drink because of the painful mouth and throat ulcers. Hospitalization is rare. See "Dehydration" section.

Contagiousness/Immunity

Hand, foot, and mouth disease is a very contagious viral illness. The virus is easily transmitted through contaminated saliva and nasal secretions. Siblings and playmates of infected children are very likely to develop it. Even parents can catch it! The incubation period after contact is 3 to 6 days. Your child is contagious approximately 2 days before and 2 to 3 days after the blisters develop. You should make your best effort to isolate your child.

Your child can return to school when his temperature returns to a normal range and the blisters are beginning to disappear. Good hand-washing techniques will substantially reduce spread of the disease.

 ## Home Care

The goals of home treatment are to relieve discomfort, provide good hydration, and return your child to normal activities as soon as possible. We ask you to first read through the entire "Home Care" section to determine which of our recommendations make the most sense for your child's current situation.

1. Diet. Avoid irritating or stinging foods such as citrus, salty, or spicy foods. Also, avoid foods that require considerable chewing. Try a soft, bland diet for the first few days and encourage plenty of clear fluids. Cold drinks, popsicles, fruit smoothies, and sherbet often work best.

2. Ulcer/blister relief.

   A. Acetaminophen or ibuprofen may at least partially relieve the discomfort from mouth ulcers. You may also try a mouth rinse with Mylanta® or Maalox®. Try 1/2 to 1 tsp. just inside the mouth after meals and snacks. These antacids coat the mouth ulcers and may reduce pain. See "OTC Medication Recommendations and Dosages" section. Chloraseptic® Throat Spray may provide some relief, as well.

   B. Hand and foot blister pain may be soothed by calamine lotion applied topically as often as necessary to relieve discomfort.

3. Acetaminophen or ibuprofen may reduce blister discomfort as well as any general muscle or joint aches that may be part of the illness. See "OTC Medication Recommendations and Dosages" section.

Integrated Therapies

(Please refer to the section on "Administering Integrated Treatments" on page 19 for guidance on using any of the therapies that follow.)

AROMATHERAPY

- An aromatherapy bath or massage with the essential oils of eucalyptus radiata and/or lavender can soothe and relax your child's anxiety and restlessness. Add 2 to 5 drops of oil to a warm bath and allow your child to soak for a comfortable period of time.

HERBAL REMEDIES (For quick reference please refer to the "Herbal Remedies List" on page 31 and the inside cover.)

- Valerian root is a mild herbal sedative that may offer some help in easing a child with significant restlessness or pain. Valerian root may be most useful at bedtime. For dosing, follow the package labeling accurately.

HOMEOPATHIC REMEDIES (For quick reference please refer to the "Homeopathic Remedies List" on page 32 and the inside cover.)

- A homeopathic remedy designed to support the defense system in viral infections may be useful. It can be taken 3 to 6 times daily when the virus is active (for example, fever, lethargy, etc.). (General Support 1)
- A homeopathic remedy designed to decrease inflammation and fever from infections may help prevent deterioration and improve the recovery time. It can be taken 3 to 6 times daily when the virus is active (for example, fever, lethargy, etc.). (General Support 2)

BACH FLOWER REMEDIES

- Rescue Remedy™ may be of use if your child is uncomfortable from the illness, stress, or anxiety. You may use 2 drops every 10 minutes to every few hours to calm restlessness as needed.
- A lukewarm bath with 10 drops of Rescue Remedy™ added to the bathwater is often very effective at relieving agitation and stress in general.

NUTRITIONALS AND SUPPLEMENTS

- Zinc

DIETARY GUIDELINES

- It is best to avoid all dairy products and citrus fruits because they may increase or thicken respiratory mucous.
- Warm foods such as soups, warm cooked grains (for example. oatmeal), and teas should be given.
- Cold foods, foods high in sugar, and fried foods should be avoided.

INTEGRATIVE SUPPORTIVE CARE

- Please read the section "Integrated Management of Respiratory Illnesses."

 ## When to Call Your Health-care Provider

Call immediately if any of the following occur:
- Your young child (less than 1 year old) has not urinated for more than 8 hours. See "Dehydration" section.
- Your older child (more than 1 year old) has not urinated in 12 hours.
- Your child has a stiff neck and/or a significant headache.
- Your child becomes confused, delirious, or hard to arouse.
- The mouth pain becomes severe with no relief from the above treatments.

Call within 24 hours if:
- The treatment options listed above are not helping.
- Your child is not better in 7 days.
- Pain control is difficult.

 ## Other Relevant Sections

Dehydration

Fever

Throat

Integrated Management of Respiratory Illnesses

HAND, FOOT & MOUTH DISEASE

🍎 Prevention

Good hand-washing is the key to reducing spread. Wash your hands thoroughly after direct contact with your child or anything your child has touched. The virus can survive on inanimate objects for several hours. Washing toys and play objects will help prevent spread of the disease.

Avoid contact with all children known to have the virus. During peak coxsackie season, avoid children who are known to be ill in any way. Children who have been exposed may not yet have symptoms. They are contagious approximately 2 days before any symptoms develop. If you have a newborn or small infant in the same house, very special attention should be paid to hand-washing.

HAY FEVER/ PERENNIAL ALLERGIES/ ENVIRONMENTAL RHINITIS

 ### Description/Physiology

Hay fever is a very common problem in children and adults. Triggers are often easy to treat when they can be identified. However, there may be dozens of triggers, which are called allergens. Allergens are small molecules our body recognizes as foreign, and its response to them is called the allergic response. Many of the allergens are seasonal (for example, weeds, pollens, grasses, etc.). Hay fever is the name of allergic symptoms from these seasonal allergens. A perennial allergy is the name for allergies caused by non-seasonal allergens (for example, dog and cat dander). Environmental rhinitis is a condition in which similar symptoms are triggered by non-allergens, such as pollutants and irritants in the air (for example, cigarette smoke, air pollution, etc.).

Hay fever, perennial allergies, and environmental rhinitis are triggered when an allergen or irritant enters the respiratory tract through the mouth, nose, or eyes. Once settled there, it irritates the mucous membranes that line these areas, creates inflammation, and stimulates the release of histamine. This inflammation and histamine release cause swelling, redness, mucous production, itching, sneezing, and watery eyes.

 ### Causes/Epidemiology

There are dozens of agents that can trigger these reactions. For hay fever, the most common are tree, grass, and weed pollen. For perennial allergies, common triggering events would include animal dander, dust, mold, feathers, etc. For environmental rhinitis, triggers could include dry air, cigarette smoke, chemical fumes, and smoke. Also, food allergies may trigger hay fever-like symptoms.

 ### Expected Course

The expected course depends on the triggering agent, the age and health of the child, other allergies present, and other accompanying symptoms.

In most instances, the symptoms of these disorders are minor annoyances that may cause a clear runny nose; itchy and puffy, watery, red eyes; a red nose;

189

sneezing; scratchy throat; and plugged ears. Other symptoms may include a cough, wheezing, constant throat clearing, sore throat, exhaustion, and sleep and feeding disruptions. Some children may suffer from nosebleeds, dark circles under the eyes, and a tendency to breathe through their mouth.

Most children respond well to home treatments described below, while others may require more aggressive treatments such as prescription medications and environmental and dietary changes.

Because many hay fever triggers are seasonal, symptoms will usually lessen and eventually disappear as the seasons change. Perennial allergies and environmental rhinitis will tend to wax and wane through the year as the triggers come and go in the environment.

It is rare for hay fever to produce secondary complications. However, because a considerable amount of mucous may be produced, there may be the possibility of secondary bacterial infections developing, such as ear infections and bacterial sinus infections. Children with asthma may experience an increase in asthma symptoms during periods of exposure to allergens.

If symptoms persist despite home and even prescription treatments, your health-care provider may recommend an evaluation by a pediatric allergist to determine exact triggers.

Contagiousness/Immunity

There are no contagious triggers for hay fever.

Home Care

The goals for treatment are primarily to provide relief for your child and to preserve sleep, appetite, and routine daily activities.

We ask you to first read through the entire "Home Care" section to select those recommendations that make the most sense for your child's particular situation.

1. Trigger. Identify the trigger and eliminate it, if possible. For example, if a cat triggers perennial allergies or mowing the lawn triggers hay fever symptoms, then avoidance of the cat or lawn-mowing is important. If certain foods trigger hay fever/allergy-like symptoms, eliminate these, as well. If the trigger cannot be easily avoided, pre-treatment with medications such as Benadryl® or Claritin® may be helpful.

2. Humidification. Run a humidifier or vaporizer in your child's room or play area as much as possible.

3. Hydration. Encourage increased clear fluid intake, which will help thin mucous and promote easy mucous flow.

4. Nasal saline rinse. Use saline nose drops made of $1/2$ teaspoon of salt and 1 cup of water or commercially available saline drops (for example, Ocean®). Put 2 drops in each nostril for several minutes and then have your child blow his nose to clear the mucous (in younger children suction away mucous with a bulb syringe). Repeat as needed 3 to 4 times per day. Nasal suctioning too frequently can cause a "rebound" with worsening congestion.

5. Medications.

   A. Antihistamines can be of great value. Please refer to the "OTC Medication Recommendations and Dosages" section. The use of OTC decongestants or decongestants/antihistamine combinations is generally not recommended because they tend to thicken the mucous and prevent its drainage. If drainage does not occur, the mucous may thicken, become colonized with bacteria, and lead to a possible secondary bacterial infection.

   B. Chromolyn sodium (NasalCrom®) is an OTC nasal medication that can significantly relieve the symptoms of hay fever and perennial allergies. For dosing, follow the package labeling accurately.

   C. If nasal congestion is significantly interfering with eating or sleeping and saline nose drops are not sufficient, you may consider using OTC phenylephrine nose drops in a strength of $1/8$% or $1/4$%. You may administer 1 to 2 drops in each nostril as needed to support eating and sleeping for a maximum of 3 doses per day for a maximum of 7 days. (Use for longer periods can result in nasal membrane dependency.)

6. Diet. Eliminate milk and dairy products when mucous production is significant.

7. Environment. Keep the house and particularly your child's room as clean as possible. Careful attention to bedding and stuffed animals is important, as they easily become reservoirs for dust, dander, and pollen.

8. Pollens. If outdoor pollens are the trigger, use air conditioning and a room air filter (such as a HEPA filter) to help remove pollens from inside the home. Have your child shower off pollens from hair and skin after coming in from outdoor play on high pollen days.

Integrated Therapies

(Please refer to the section on "Administering Integrated Treatments" on page 19 for guidance on using any of the therapies that follow.)

AROMATHERAPY

- Add 2 drops each of the essential oils of eucalyptus radiata and lavender to 1 to 2 teaspoons of olive oil and rub on your child's chest to soothe a cough or congestion from hay fever.
- An aromatherapy bath or massage with the essential oils of eucalyptus radiata and/or lavender can soothe and relax your child and soothe a cough or congestion from hay fever. Add 2 to 5 drops of oil to a warm bath and allow your child to soak for a comfortable period of time.

HERBAL REMEDIES (For quick reference please refer to the "Herbal Remedies List" on page 31 and the inside cover.)

- Valerian root is a mild herbal sedative that may offer some help in easing a child with significant restlessness or itching. Valerian root may be most useful at bedtime. For dosing, follow the package labeling accurately.

HOMEOPATHIC REMEDIES (For quick reference please refer to the "Homeopathic Remedies List" on page 32 and the inside cover.)

- A homeopathic remedy designed to help minimize the impact of allergies from any cause may be helpful with hay fever and perennial allergies. It can be taken 2 to 6 times daily for allergy symptoms. (Respiratory 7)
- A homeopathic remedy nasal spray designed to minimize the runny nose and congestion associated with hay fever and allergies may be helpful. It can be taken 2 to 4 times daily for allergy symptoms. (Respiratory 11)
- A homeopathic remedy designed to relieve red, itching eyes and skin, especially when caused by allergic reactions, may be helpful. It can be taken 3 to 6 times daily until the itching resolves. (Skin 3)
- A homeopathic remedy designed to minimize nasal congestion and mucous, especially when associated with environmental irritants, may be useful. It can be taken 2 to 3 times daily while there is nasal congestion. (Respiratory 3)

BACH FLOWER REMEDIES

- Rescue Remedy™ may be of use if your child is uncomfortable from the illness, stress, or anxiety. You may use 2 drops every 10 minutes to every few hours to calm restlessness as needed.
- A lukewarm bath with 10 drops of Rescue Remedy™ added to the bathwater is often very effective at relieving agitation and stress in general.

NUTRITIONALS AND SUPPLEMENTS

- Vitamin C

DIETARY GUIDELINES

- Avoid any food that you suspect your child is sensitive to.
- Avoid mucous-forming foods, especially all dairy products and citrus fruits and their juices.
- An important aspect of dietary management of allergies is good fluid intake. You may use the following table as a general guideline for water in addition to normal fluid intake:

AGE	OUNCES OF WATER PER DAY
2 to 5 years old	12 to 18 ounces
5 to 12 years old	18 to 24 ounces
13 and up	32 to 48 ounces

 When to Call Your Health-care Provider

Hay fever is not an emergency. If there are acute and very severe allergy symptoms that develop, this is not hay fever. Instead, it is possible that a serious allergic reaction, characterized by wheezing, increased work of breathing, color changes, swelling of the throat, and extreme agitation may develop. This could be a far more serious condition, called an anaphylactic reaction. This is an emergency and requires immediate treatment. You should call 911.

Call within 24 hours if:
- Hay fever symptoms are worsening.
- Hay fever symptoms are no better after 3 days of the above treatments.
- Your child develops wheezing.
- Your child is unable to sleep restfully.
- Symptoms are disrupting your child's daily routine.

- Hives are present.
- Your child has a significant sore throat, especially if there has been a strep exposure.
- The cough takes a turn for the worse, especially accompanied by a fever.

Other Relevant Sections

Asthma

Colds

Conjunctivitis

Cough

Eczema

Hives

Nosebleeds

Throat

Prevention

Prevention of hay fever requires careful observation and identification of its trigger(s). Once pinpointed, avoid contact with the offending agent or agents. Anticipate venues where there may be these expected exposures, such as a state fair with animal danders. This is true for exposure to foods, animal dander, plants, and flowers. Avoid cigarette smoke as much as possible.

To further avoid exposure to pollens and outdoor molds, stay inside with windows closed during seasons that are the most problematic. Pollen counts are usually higher in the afternoon. Air conditioning is preferable to evaporative cooling. Vacuum carpets 1 to 2 times per week. Use a HEPA filter or double bag in the vacuum. Consider replacing carpet with vinyl, tile, or wood flooring. Use of air filtration systems or HEPA room air purifiers can be helpful, as can regular duct cleaning. Use only properly cleaned humidifiers and take note if humidifier use increases your child's symptoms.

Allergy treatments can help enhance lifestyle by allowing more liberal exposure to the outdoors. A consultation with your health-care provider may provide additional treatment options for your child's comfort.

Description/Physiology

A headache is a relatively common complaint in children. Most headaches are benign, infrequent, and easy to treat; however, in some children, headaches may occur frequently and a chronic pattern may emerge. The majority of headaches will disappear following minimal intervention and the passage of time. Headaches tend to run in families and are more common in girls than boys.

Children describe headaches in many ways, depending on the age of the child and the type of headache. Of course, infants and toddlers cannot specifically describe the features of their headache, but they may show irritability, agitation, sleep loss, poor appetite, fever, and vomiting. Some infants will rub their eyes, pull their hair, shake their head, and moan inconsolably. It is almost impossible to localize the exact site of a headache in this age group. At the same time, an infant or toddler will likely have other symptoms besides the headache that are part of the overall illness.

Older children can help by giving us more information about the headache. They may give us descriptions of the pain like throbbing, sharp, dull, a tight band around the head, and pounding. They may tell us exactly where the pain is, when it started, what triggered it, other accompanying symptoms, and if they have had other similar headaches.

Severity of headache pain can be thought of in 3 ways:

1. Mild: Child barely mentions the headache, and it rarely, if ever, interferes with daily activities.

2. Moderate: Child complains of the headache, and it does interfere to some extent with daily routine.

3. Severe: The child may be in extreme pain, inconsolable, or agitated. He may awaken from sleep with the headache.

 Causes/Epidemiology

It is beyond the scope of this handbook to fully discuss all the possible types of headaches and their precise characteristics, expected course, and treatments. We will, however, provide you with general principles of common headache types in children and guidelines for their treatment.

There are many different causes of headaches. A careful history and description of all the features of the headache will help your health-care provider establish a diagnosis and, in turn, provide specific guidelines for treatment.

Here are some of the primary causes of headaches in children:

1. Muscular tension headaches: Tension headaches, especially in the muscles of the back of the head and neck.

2. Vascular headaches: Migraine or cluster headaches or headaches from increased blood pressure. Dehydration-triggered headaches can be included in this category.

3. Traction headaches: Headaches after head trauma; post-concussion headaches.

4. Inflammatory/infection-triggered headaches: Earache, sinus infections, meningitis, encephalitis.

5. Headaches triggered by visual problems/eye strain and squinting in bright light.

6. Headaches triggered by allergies, including food allergies.

7. Psychological stress and emotional triggers.

8. Other less common causes of headaches include reactions to medications; poisonings; toxin exposures such as carbon monoxide; very rarely, a brain tumor; and skipping meals, which may be related to blood sugar levels.

When evaluating the cause of headaches, we distinguish between acute headaches, such as those associated with an illness, infection, tension, or trauma, versus chronic or recurrent headaches, which are more likely associated with migraines, allergies, chronic sinusitis, or eye problems.

Acute headaches associated with an infection, fever, earache, trauma, etc., are rarely serious and generally respond to acetaminophen or ibuprofen along with appropriate treatment of the underlying problem. Many acute headaches are simply the result of the tension and stress of the underlying illness. Acute headaches can occasionally reach severe levels of pain. This is usually when the headache is triggered by a more serious cause, such as a head injury or meningitis. Children with meningitis will usually have fever, a very stiff neck, lethargy or extreme agitation, and vomiting.

Chronic headaches caused by stress, tension, allergies, or visual changes need further evaluation. Before calling your health-care provider, please keep a week's diary of the headache and all its features. Some important details to record in your diary are:

- The time of day the headache occurs.
- How long the headache lasts.

- How severe the headaches are (use a scale of 1 as mild to 10 as severe).
- What, if anything, makes the headache better or worse (for example, movement, light, noise, medications, etc.).
- What other symptoms are associated with the headache (for example, dizziness, stomachache, vomiting, confusion, blurred vision, etc.).
- Where the headache is located and the quality of the pain (for example, sharp, dull, constant, intermittent, pounding, or throbbing).
- Whether there is an allergy history or any environmental changes (car trips, sunlight exposure, food triggers, emotional upset, serious life transitions, significant altitude changes, etc.).

 ## Expected Course

The course of each headache depends largely on its trigger and the age of the child. Most acute headaches have an obvious trigger—for example, head injury, fatigue, or the flu. Acute headaches generally respond well to the usual treatments listed below. There is no "average" length of time for a headache, but the majority will resolve within 1 to 2 hours of onset and/or treatment.

Headaches are considered chronic when they recur for more than 3 to 4 weeks. Again, identifying the trigger is the key to predicting the severity and duration of these headaches. A migraine headache is a common example of a chronic headache. It is characterized by a severe, usually pounding headache, often one-sided in nature, which may be brought on by a predictable trigger (light, smell, a menstrual period, stress). It is often preceded by a visual disturbance or "aura" and there may be nausea and vomiting. There is no specific duration to these headaches, either, and they also often resolve quickly with treatment. However, they may continue to recur until the underlying diagnosis is treated.

If your child develops chronic headaches, he may be referred for evaluation to a pediatric neurologist. Careful record-keeping is invaluable, as the diagnosis is often made by history, since most children with headaches will have a totally normal physical and neurological exam.

 ## Contagiousness/Immunity

The headache itself is not contagious; however, if there is a viral or bacterial cause of the headache, these infectious agents are certainly contagious. Whether they produce a headache in a newly infected child depends on the child, the virus, and the body's unique response to the infection.

HEADACHES

🏠 Home Care

Not all headaches will respond to the suggestions below, but most will. We offer you guidelines here for comfort. Relieving the headache and restoring your child's comfort are the primary, immediate objectives. Once this is accomplished, your health-care provider can investigate triggers and recommend prevention and avoidance techniques. More aggressive treatments may be necessary to cure the underlying cause, including prescription medications. And a combination of therapies may be required for full relief.

We ask you to read through the entire "Home Care" section first to determine which recommendations make the most sense for your child's current situation.

1. Hydration: Many children are simply under-hydrated. Kids often forget to drink water before and while engaged in sports and outdoor activities. Gently re-hydrate your child with clear liquids and then take measures to ensure he stays well-hydrated in the future. Milk is probably best avoided initially, unless it is the only fluid your child will take.

2. Head position: Elevate your child's head above the heart level while he is sleeping. This maneuver may help relieve the throbbing sensation of a headache that is worsened by lying flat.

3. Ibuprofen or acetaminophen: Ibuprofen is probably the better agent for headache relief. These medicines may work best if started early in the course of a headache. See "OTC Medication Recommendations and Dosages" section.

4. Environment: A quiet, dark room may help. Reduce unnecessary noise, sunlight, your child's activity, and general commotion around your child.

5. For older children, quiet meditation or relaxation exercises may be advised.

6. Consistent nutrition is important. Some children are prone to headaches if they eat erratically or eat too many sugary foods. Many children with headaches do best with 3 consistent meals and several healthy snacks evenly spaced throughout the day.

7. Because a food allergy may trigger a headache, if you detect a headache triggered by a specific food, eliminate that food from your child's diet.

8. Gentle scalp and forehead massage with warm massage oil may help. Concentrate on the temples. A general body massage may relieve tension.

9. A cool washcloth across the forehead may help.

10. Pay close attention to potential dietary causes. Caffeine causes headaches in many children who drink sodas or other caffeine-containing products. Artificial sweeteners, MSG, and nitrite food preservatives have also been associated with causing headaches.

 ## Integrated Therapies

(Please refer to the section on "Administering Integrated Treatments" on page 19 for guidance on using any of the therapies that follow.)

AROMATHERAPY

- An aromatherapy bath or massage with the essential oil lavender can soothe and relax your child's anxiety and restlessness. Add 2 to 5 drops of oil to a warm bath and allow your child to soak for a comfortable period of time.
- Rub one drop of peppermint and/or lavender essential oil on the temple (careful to avoid the eyes) and/or the back of the neck.

HERBAL REMEDIES (For quick reference please refer to the "Herbal Remedies List" on page 31 and the inside cover.)

- Valerian root is a mild herbal sedative that may help a child with significant restlessness, thus relieving the headache. Valerian root may be most useful at bedtime. For dosing, follow the package labeling accurately.

HOMEOPATHIC REMEDIES (For quick reference please refer to the "Homeopathic Remedies List" on page 32 and the inside cover.)

- A homeopathic remedy designed to relax muscle spasm may be useful to help relieve the pain of a tension headache. It can be given 3 to 8 times per day as needed for relief of tension. (Pain 1)
- A homeopathic remedy designed to soothe restlessness, which can be associated with a headache, may be useful. It may be taken every 15 to 30 minutes for 1 hour or until the restlessness subsides. (Pain 2)
- A homeopathic remedy designed to help relieve a headache and its symptoms may help in resolving and preventing headaches. It can be taken every 15 to 60 minutes during a headache or 2 times daily for prevention. (Pain 3)

BACH FLOWER REMEDIES

- Rescue Remedy™ may be of use if your child is uncomfortable from the

illness, stress, or anxiety. You may use 2 drops every 10 minutes to every few hours to calm restlessness as needed.
- A lukewarm bath with 10 drops of Rescue Remedy™ added to the bathwater is often very effective at relieving agitation and stress in general.

NUTRITIONALS AND SUPPLEMENTS
- Magnesium
- Probiotics

DIETARY GUIDELINES
- Eliminate caffeine and sugar from the diet.
- Your child should drink extra water to ensure good hydration. You may use the following table as a general guideline for water in addition to normal fluid intake:

AGE	OUNCES OF WATER PER DAY
2 to 5 years old	12 to 18 ounces
5 to 12 years old	18 to 24 ounces
13 and up	32 to 48 ounces

 When to Call Your Health-care Provider

Call immediately if any of the following occur:
- The headache is associated with repeated vomiting, significant behavior changes (disorientation, amnesia, confusion, combativeness), and worsening pain.
- The headache is associated with a rigid, stiff neck.
- After head injury, the headache worsens.
- There has been no improvement in the headache 24 hours after head injury.
- Your child is increasingly difficult to awaken or is unconscious.
- Your child has an unsteady walk or is significantly off-balance.
- Your child suffers the loss of normal nervous system function—for example, he is unable to move an extremity or has slurred speech.
- There is loss of sensation anywhere on the body, especially the extremities.
- There is loss of vision or blurred vision in one or both eyes.
- The pain is severe or incapacitating.

Call within 24 hours if:
- Your child awakens in the middle of the night with a headache.
- A chronic pattern of headaches develops over 2 to 4 weeks or longer.
- Your child appears to be dehydrated. See "Dehydration" section.

Other Relevant Sections

Colds

Dehydration

Earache/Ear Infection

Fever

Head Injury

Influenza

Sinus Infection

Stress

Throat

Vomiting

Prevention

Prevention of a headache is best determined by its cause. For example, if specific allergies cause headaches, attention should be paid to avoid those allergen triggers.

Dehydration is a common cause of headaches, especially in adolescents. Prevention here means supplying your child with plenty of fluids, especially before and during exercise and outdoor activity. You may also need to frequently remind your child to drink. Children engaged in focused activities often forget to keep up with their hydration.

Migraine headaches may have common triggers, including smells, bright lights, a new or increased stress, caffeine, a menstrual period, and certain foods. Knowing these triggers allows you to craft an environment as free of these inciting agents as possible.

Viral- and bacterial-triggered headaches are prevented through conscious avoidance of other children known to be ill. This is understandably difficult in all circumstances, but during known epidemics, you are encouraged to avoid contact with locations where large numbers of children congregate.

For a child prone to tension headaches, pay close attention to his environment in order to intervene when stress, tension, and unexpected circumstances cause your child to be overwhelmed or agitated. Please see "Stress" section. If stress is a cause, observe your child's environment and life carefully and act to eliminate all stressful triggers. Again, your child might respond well to daily relaxation exercises or even daily massage, especially at the end of a stressful day. Your tender, loving care works wonders!

If you feel that your child is suffering from headaches due to extreme stress (such as with a divorce, school issues, etc.), please talk to your health-care provider for further suggestions on stress management.

Avoid cigarette smoke exposure for those children with smell sensitivities. This may be true for other smells for which you will identify a pattern of headache trigger (strong perfumes, cleaning solvents, certain foods).

Teach your child to eat meals regularly and consider consistent snacks if it appears that the headache is caused by hunger. Be sure to include a protein at each meal and snack to provide your child with a consistent energy level.

Description/Physiology

Head injuries are a common experience throughout childhood. Fortunately, most head injuries are just simple bumps to the head that cause soft tissue swelling and bruising. Severe head injuries are much less common but can be very frightening, and may require prompt medical attention.

The immediate goals after a head injury are to assess the severity of the situation and any danger to your child. Some of the factors to consider in this assessment include:

- the type of injury
- what part of the head has been injured
- loss of consciousness or the occurrence of a seizure
- presence of vomiting
- the degree of general discomfort following the injury
- the height of a fall
- the presence of cuts and bruises
- the presence and severity of headache
- possible injury to the neck
- how long and what it took for your child to stop crying

There can be several types of head injury with varying degrees of danger, including:

1. Injuries to the scalp only (cuts, bruises, and swelling).

2. Skull injuries (bone bruises or fractures of the bone).

3. Concussion (usually a brief period of disorientation, loss of memory, or even brief loss of consciousness).

4. Trauma directly to the brain associated with worsening neurologic symptoms such as inability to speak, walk, think clearly, arouse, and interact with you.

Causes/Epidemiology

Common head injuries may occur with falls, direct blows to the head, tumbles down stairways, etc. Toddlers may bump their heads a few times per day by falls to the ground or against objects, or sometimes as a behavioral response to injury or frustration (temper tantrums, breath-holding spells, or head banging).

HEAD INJURY

Older children may suffer head injuries from sports activities, from bicycle injuries (whether a helmet is worn is not), from a direct blow to the head in a fight, because of clumsiness and inattention, and so forth. Head injuries may occur in motor vehicle accidents, as well.

 ## Expected Course

Most head injuries are mild and children recover quickly. Don't be surprised by the quick appearance of the characteristic "goose egg" on the scalp or forehead. These "goose egg" swellings can be remarkably large and immediate, especially on the forehead. With proper treatment, head swelling will slowly resolve, but there may remain a bruise and a firm lump under the skin for a number of weeks. Headache from head injury usually is short-lived. Again, proper treatment and distraction likely will bring pain under control within an hour of the injury. Many children may be dizzy and drowsy for several hours to a day after a mild head injury.

Loss of consciousness at the time of the injury is very serious. You should call 911 if your child does not regain consciousness within 1 minute. Sometimes "the wind is knocked out" of your child or there may be a "breath-holding spell" following a head injury. Your child may be drowsy, a bit disoriented, and "spacey" for a few minutes, but should slowly regain full consciousness. The headache may start immediately and persist for several hours, eventually resolving within 24 hours.

Persistent or worsening headache can be a sign of a more significant injury. A skull fracture is very unlikely but does occur in 1 percent to 2 percent of head injuries. Loss of consciousness some time after the injury is also worrisome. Vomiting may occur once or twice after any head injury, and, in general, 1 to 2 vomiting episodes are acceptable. However, if more than 2 vomiting episodes occur, either right after the event or any time within the first 24 hours, you should notify your health-care provider. Watch for signs of progressive lethargy, difficulty arousing your child, disorientation, and amnesia.

 ## Contagiousness/Immunity

This section does not apply to head injury.

Home Care

The goal for home care is to relieve the pain and establish the severity of the injury. Your calm demeanor will go a long way to reassure your child that everything is all right. Meantime, your careful observation of your child will help determine whether a more significant injury has occurred. The following home treatments generally are sufficient to handle the problem. The more severe symptoms require a more thorough evaluation and therapy.

We ask you to first read through this entire "Home Care" section and select those recommendations that make the most sense for your child's current situation.

1. Acetaminophen or ibuprofen will often provide relief within one hour of their administration. Please refer to "OTC Medication Recommendations and Dosages" section.

2. Apply an ice pack to the swelling for ten minutes every half-hour for several applications until the swelling subsides. A bag of frozen peas often works well.

3. As much as possible, limit physical activity for 24 hours.

4. Elevate the head of the bed with an extra pillow during sleep and rest. This head-up position helps minimize swelling.

5. Use a very bland diet and give no dairy products or formula for 24 hours. Give small sips of clear liquids initially to see if vomiting occurs. If all goes well, you may resume a normal diet within several hours.

6. It is common for your child to fall asleep following the stress of a head injury. You may let your child nap, with his head elevated, for about 1 to 2 hours after the injury. Let your child sleep, but arouse him every 60 minutes to ensure that he is easily aroused. If you cannot arouse your child, call your health-care provider immediately.

7. Local wound care may be necessary for superficial cuts and scrapes. Wash the area gently with soap and water and apply an antibacterial cream.

8. When there has been a significant head injury, we suggest that you arouse your child at your own bedtime and again once during the night. Arousal in this instance means to be sure that your child can be sufficiently awakened to answer questions, take a sip of water, and interact with you. You do not need to awaken your child every hour through the night. If you cannot arouse your child, call your health-care provider immediately.

9. You do not need to check your child's pupils. This is a common myth and of minimal value. Unequal pupils are a sign of such serious deterioration that there will be several other more obvious symptoms that present long before the pupils become unequal, such as loss of consciousness, abnormal breathing, etc.

10. After a head injury, please avoid medications that may cause drowsiness (for example, Benadryl®, valerian root, etc.).

 ## Integrated Therapies

(Please refer to the section on "Administering Integrated Treatments" on page 19 for guidance on using any of the therapies that follow.)

AROMATHERAPY

- An aromatherapy bath or massage with the essential oil lavender can soothe and relax your child's anxiety and restlessness. Add 2 to 5 drops of oil to a warm bath and allow your child to soak for a comfortable period of time.
- Rub one drop of lavender essential oil on the temple (careful to avoid the eyes) and/or the back of the neck.

HOMEOPATHIC REMEDIES (For quick reference please refer to the "Homeopathic Remedies List" on page 32 and the inside cover.)

- A homeopathic remedy designed to speed the body's recovery from injury may help minimize swelling and inflammation. It may be taken as 1 tablet or 4 drops—3 to 6 times a day until the injury is resolved. (General Support 4)

BACH FLOWER REMEDIES

- Rescue Remedy™ may be of use if your child is uncomfortable from the illness, stress, or anxiety. You may use 2 drops every 10 minutes to every few hours to calm restlessness as needed.
- A lukewarm bath with 10 drops of Rescue Remedy™ added to the bathwater is often very effective at relieving agitation and stress in general.

When to Call Your Health-care Provider

Call immediately if any of the following occur:
- A loss of consciousness at the time of the head injury.
- A change in your child's level of alertness. For example, if he becomes progressively more disoriented, lethargic, or has trouble speaking to you.
- If there is a reason to suspect a neck injury, do not move your child until medical help arrives.
- Marked, unsteady gait or poor coordination, especially if this poor balance worsens.
- Vomiting 1 or 2 times is common. If vomiting persists for more than 2 hours beyond the injury or begins again several hours after the injury, call your health-care provider.
- A headache is expected following a head injury, but it usually subsides within 1 to 2 hours after treatment. If the headache increases in severity, call your health-care provider. Small children who can't complain of their pain may be very restless and irritable with a headache. Sleep and feeding may be significantly disrupted.
- Bleeding that won't stop after even 10 minutes of continuous direct pressure. (See "First Aid—Cuts and Abrasions" section.)
- Your child's skin is split open and probably needs stitches (greater than $^1/_8$" wide).
- The accident was a severe one involving great force—for example, a fall down a stairway, a fall from a significant height, head trauma in a car accident.
- Your child's crying lasts more than 20 to 30 minutes after the injury.
- Your child has a seizure.
- Your child is very disoriented, confused, or has amnesia after the injury.
- Your child's speech is slurred.
- Your child's vision is blurred or double.

Call within 24 hours if:
- The headache persists for more than 24 hours.
- Balance and movement are not better by 24 hours.
- Signs of dehydration develop. See "Dehydration" section.
- You suspect that your child has a mild concussion.

HEAD INJURY

 Other Relevant Sections

Dehydration

Headache

Vomiting

First Aid—Cuts and Abrasions

 Prevention

Even under constant surveillance, it is impossible to prevent all head injuries—for example, head bumps on furniture, blows by siblings, and headers while running. You can't be everywhere at once to cushion a fall or a blow. You do the best you can!

Infants should never be left alone on high surfaces. NEVER place your car seat/baby seat on a countertop or table. Keep the side rails of the crib up at all times. Baby walkers are a hazard in the active child. Don't leave your baby in a shopping cart unattended for even a few seconds.

In toddlers, prevention of head injury is a challenge. Fortunately, the distance they fall is usually short (their own height!), and this age group is resilient. Your home should be fully safety-proofed, particularly against the most worrisome injuries such as falls down stairs, off heights, etc. This means placement of safety gates at the top of stairs. Keep your stairway free of objects that you might trip over while carrying your baby.

In all children, HELMET USE for tricycles, bicycles, skiing, skateboard, and rollerblading is mandatory and can be life-saving. Buckle up children of all ages, either in their car seats or age-appropriate restraints. Watch your children during outside play until they are at least 5 or 6 years of age.

Children with a significant head injury during sporting events should be sidelined immediately. Head injury, coupled with dehydration induced by intense physical activity, is a bad combination. All children and adolescents with loss of consciousness must be sidelined immediately. They may return to play only after a 1-week period of observation, no activity, and clearance from a medical professional. After a concussion, the brain is much more susceptible to injury from mild impact.

Safety instruction regarding crossing streets, retrieving balls, and staying out of alleys is essential. We do not encourage trampolines, but if your child does use one, provide constant supervision, and permit only one person to jump at a time.

Description/Physiology

Hives are a common skin rash characterized by raised pink or red spots, sometimes with pale, raised centers called welts. Hives vary in size and shape and may be an inch to several inches wide. They are almost always itchy. Hives may come and go over a period of minutes, hours, or even days. They may occur anywhere on the body. It may be difficult to trace the exact cause of hives unless an obvious trigger is present.

Causes/Epidemiology

Hives are caused by the release of the body's own histamine into the skin in response to an inciting agent. Histamine release can be triggered by any of the following events:

- An allergic reaction to new foods, cosmetics, clothing, plants, detergents, and certain soaps.
- Allergic reactions to medication, especially antibiotics. This is even more likely if your child has had a previous exposure to the same antibiotic or a related member of that antibiotic family.
- As a part of an allergic reaction to an insect or spider bite, bee sting, or direct contact with a specific animal.
- In association with a strep infection. Hives may be the only symptom you will see with strep.
- In association with some viral infections, even if there are no other symptoms. In some viral infections, hives may be the most obvious manifestation of the virus.
- Sometimes hives are triggered by cold temperature.

Expected Course

The course of hives depends on its triggering agent. Mild reactions may begin with a few scattered patches of hives that may disappear over several hours to a day without treatment. If there is a significant allergic reaction or bite, the rash may develop rapidly, be more generalized across the body, and last for several days to even weeks. Hives may appear on one part of the body, and then disappear, only to reappear elsewhere. Hives may also appear and remain in that location for the duration of the rash.

HIVES

Hives associated with allergic reactions may also accompany symptoms such as runny nose, itchy eyes, scratchy throat, sneezing, and even wheezing. Most mild hive reactions caused by allergies respond well to simple treatments listed below.

Significant allergic reactions may also include increased work of breathing, wheezing, color changes, facial swelling, lethargy, and agitation. The most profound allergic reaction is called anaphylaxis. Anaphylaxis will usually begin with an allergic reaction and generally will progress rapidly. While it is quite rare, it represents a true medical emergency. There is the potential for swollen oral tissues to eventually close off the airway. Profound and life-threatening reactions may be seen with nuts, shellfish, insect bites, and some medications.

Some children have recurrent bouts with hives. These are mostly children with allergy causes.

Contagiousness/Immunity

Hives themselves are not transmitted from one person to another. However, infectious causes, primarily viruses or strep, can be passed from one child to another.

Home Care

The primary goals for treating hives are to relieve discomfort and itching. We ask you to first read through the entire "Home Care" section to select which of our recommendations make the most sense for your child's current situation.

1. Cool baths 1 to 2 times daily. Consider oatmeal added to the bath.

2. Soak a flannel-type pajama in water and wring it out well. Have your child put on these pajamas and then put on a dry pair over them. The slow evaporation will cool the skin and thus relieve itching.

3. Antihistamines such as Benadryl®. Please see "OTC Medication Recommendations and Dosages" section. An antihistamine will not cure the root cause of hives, but it will reduce their number and intensity, as well as relieve itching.
   Note: Benadryl® may make your child somewhat drowsy.

4. If hives are not caused by a food allergy or medication reaction, your child should have a strep test to rule out a strep infection. This rapid strep test can be done during routine office hours.

5. Topical treatment with calamine lotion can soothe the itch. If you are using oral Benadryl®, be careful not to use topical agents that also contain Benadryl® (diphenhydramine) because doing so can increase the sedative side effect.

6. If cold temperature is the trigger, immediately warm your child and avoid cold exposure as much as possible.

7. Remove the offending allergen when identified. For example, wool clothing may produce hives in a susceptible child.

 Integrated Therapies

(Please refer to the section on "Administering Integrated Treatments" on page 19 for guidance on using any of the therapies that follow.)

AROMATHERAPY

- An aromatherapy bath or massage with the essential oil lavender can soothe and relax your child's anxiety and restlessness. Add 2 to 5 drops of oil to a warm bath and allow your child to soak for a comfortable period of time.

HERBAL REMEDIES (For quick reference please refer to the "Herbal Remedies List" on page 31 and the inside cover.)

- Aloe vera or calendula applied topically can reduce itching and soothe irritated skin. They are available in gel, lotion, or cream. For dosing, follow the package labeling accurately.
- Valerian root is a mild herbal sedative that may offer some help in easing a child with significant restlessness or itching. Valerian root may be most useful at bedtime. For dosing, follow the package labeling accurately.

HOMEOPATHIC REMEDIES (For quick reference please refer to the "Homeopathic Remedies List" on page 32 and the inside cover.)

- A homeopathic cream designed to soothe inflamed, irritated, or itching skin may be useful. It can be applied directly to the infected area 3 times a day. (Skin 1)
- A homeopathic remedy designed to relieve red, itching skin, especially when caused by a skin reaction such as insect bites or irritants may be helpful. It can be taken 3 to 6 times daily until the itching and redness resolve. (Skin 3)

BACH FLOWER REMEDIES

- Rescue Remedy™ may be of use if your child is uncomfortable from the illness, stress, or anxiety. You may use 2 drops every 10 minutes to every few hours to calm restlessness as needed.
- A lukewarm bath with 10 drops of Rescue Remedy™ added to the bathwater is often very effective at relieving agitation and stress in general.

NUTRITIONALS AND SUPPLEMENTS

- Vitamin C

DIETARY GUIDELINES

- Avoid any food that you suspect your child is sensitive to.
- Pay close attention to hydration, especially if there is a fever present, as inflamed skin increases body fluid loss, thus predisposing the child to dehydration.

 When to Call Your Health-care Provider

Call immediately if any of the following occur:

- There is any difficulty with swallowing, excessive drooling, or problems with breathing (wheezing, increased work of breathing, etc.)
- Hives become dark purple, painful, or associated with high fever.
- Despite the above measures the intensity of the itch worsens and becomes intolerable.
- Your child is increasingly more lethargic.

Call within 24 hours if:

- Hives have begun while your child is on a medication, including antibiotics. Stop the medication until you have spoken with your health-care provider.
- Hives persist for longer than one week.
- Hives are associated with mild swelling of the hands, feet, or lips.

 Other Relevant Sections

Colds
Eczema
Throat (Strep)

Prevention

Knowing the trigger of hives is the best weapon for prevention. Unfortunately, many triggers are unanticipated and may never be known. If the hives are short-lived, it probably doesn't matter. If the trigger is not obvious and the hives have lasted longer than a week, start documenting symptom details in a notebook, with such observations as time and date of onset, what activity may have preceded the onset, location of the hives, other general symptoms, new foods, and medications. Since viral infections often cause a hive-like rash, prevention techniques directed against the spread of viral infections, such as careful hand-washing, covering one's face while coughing, etc., can reduce viral spread.

When a medication trigger (such as an antibiotic) is known, it is important to carefully review all future medications before you give them to your child to be sure that they do not contain that medication trigger. It is always helpful to keep a list of specific medication allergies close at hand for quick and accurate reference, including when you travel. The same medication may have different names, so be sure to ask your health-care provider or pharmacist if the prescribed medication contains the drug to which your child is allergic. With severe allergic reactions you may want to consider a medical identification bracelet declaring the allergic medication.

IMPETIGO

Description/Physiology

Impetigo occurs fairly frequently in children. Because it is often on the face, the diagnosis may be made early and treatment initiated with little delay. Impetigo is characterized by small sores usually near the nose or mouth. The sores can extend inside the nostril as well. The lesions may also appear at any location on the skin where the defenses have been broken down by a disruption such as trauma, scratching, a bite, or sunburn.

Causes/Epidemiology

Impetigo is a superficial infection of the skin caused primarily by bacteria, usually either streptococcus or staphylococcus. While it occurs all year round, it is more common in the summer months. Rashes, skin scrapes, splinters, and insect bites may create a break in the normal skin barrier, allowing the bacteria, which live on the skin's surface, to invade into the deeper layers of the skin below.

Expected Course

These sores begin as small, red bumps that may develop into cloudy blisters, which often ooze yellowish, clear fluid. This clear, yellow fluid may turn to pus drainage. Underneath these blisters is very inflamed, tender skin. Eventually a soft, honey-colored crust covers these sores. The sores can by very itchy and sometimes painful.

On occasion, the infection begins inside the nose and may extend outside the nostril. The lesions may also start in the moist corners of the mouth. Sores may appear on the arms and legs, as well, likely triggered by a scrape, scratch, or bite.

With proper treatment, your child's skin will be completely healed in approximately one week. Some minor discoloration may remain in the healing area for up to 2 to 4 months.

Contagiousness/Immunity

Impetigo is mildly contagious. It is spread generally by contaminated fingers, either those of the child himself or those of a caretaker or parent. Thus, careful hand-washing remains the key to prevent its spread. Impetigo is spread to sites elsewhere on the body by scratching with contaminated fingers. It cannot be spread in the air.

Your child may return to school or daycare after 24 hours of antibiotic treatment. Although the lesions certainly will not have cleared completely within 24 hours, the active bacterial infection has been reduced to a non-contagious level by the antibiotic after 24 hours of treatment. If your child has facial lesions, you may want to keep him away from other children for an extra day or so until the facial lesions begin to heal. They will do so quickly after treatment is begun. Lesions elsewhere, and on less obvious locations on the body, can be covered by a loose gauze bandage or BAND-AID®.

Impetigo has a tendency to occur more than once in the same child. Thus, no immunity is conferred to the infected child by having had impetigo. Some children may have several bouts within the same year.

Other conditions may look like impetigo in its early stages; these include ringworm, eczema, and herpes type 1 infection. These three diseases have very different features, treatments, and courses. A health-care provider's exam can differentiate them in most instances.

 ## Home Care

The primary goals for treatment are to reduce discomfort and itching and to prevent spread of the disease. We ask you to first read through the entire "Home Care" section and select those recommendations that make the most sense for your child's current situation.

1. Antibiotics. Most children with impetigo require antibiotic therapy. Your health-care provider may ask you to bring your child to the office to confirm the diagnosis, and then they may prescribe an antibiotic. Mild cases, caught early, may respond to a topical antibiotic such as Bactroban Cream® or Neosporin®. In most cases, impetigo is treated with an oral antibiotic. Be sure to give the antibiotic for the full course recommended, even if the lesions have cleared, to help minimize the chance of recurrence and/or the development of germ resistance to antibiotics.

2. Removing the scabs. Strep or staph bacteria live on the inflamed skin tissues just underneath the crusty scabs. Until these crusts are removed, antibiotic ointment cannot penetrate to the bacteria to kill them. These crusts can be soaked off, using hydrogen peroxide rinses or even gentle soap and water. After soaking, these lesions may require a gentle rub to remove the scab, but avoid vigorous scrubbing, which only further irritates the tender skin underneath. There may be a bit of bleeding with crust removal.

3. Soap. The area should be washed 2 to 3 times daily with an antibacterial soap, each time before applying the ointment (see below). Again, gentle washing with minimal rubbing and a thorough rinsing of remaining soap is recommended. A daily bath is recommended.

4. Antibiotic ointment. After the crust has been removed, antibiotic ointment should be applied to the inflamed surface 2 to 3 times daily. We recommend Neosporin® or Bacitracin ointment, both available over-the-counter, or your health-care provider may prescribe Bactroban Cream®, which is a prescription. The ointment itself can help moisten the crust and facilitate its removal. Apply this antibiotic ointment until the lesions have completely disappeared and for 2 days beyond that time.

5. If itching is intense and none of the above measures help, consider a dose of Benadryl®. See "OTC Medication Recommendations and Dosages" section.

6. Encourage your child to avoid picking or scratching the scabs. This can be difficult to enforce in young children. It may also help to regularly trim and scrub fingernails to help prevent spreading the infection.

 ## Integrated Therapies

(Please refer to the section on "Administering Integrated Treatments" on page 19 for guidance on using any of the therapies that follow.)

AROMATHERAPY

- Add 4 drops of lavender essential oil to the tea tree oil wash (see below) if the skin itches.

HERBAL REMEDIES (For quick reference please refer to the "Herbal Remedies List" on page 31 and the inside cover.)

- Tea tree oil, for topical use only, has a natural antibiotic and antifungal effect. If the skin appears to become infected, use the tea tree oil 2 to 3 times a day. As a preventive it can be used 2 to 3 times a week. A tea tree oil skin wash, gel, or cream is best as the full strength oil is too strong for your child's skin. To make tea tree oil skin wash, add 10 drops of therapeutic grade tea tree oil to 1 ounce of purified water and apply 3 times a day with a cotton pad or from a spray bottle.

- Aloe vera or calendula applied topically can reduce itching and soothe irritated skin and so may be useful in healing the skin after the infection responds to therapy. They are available in gel, lotion, or cream. For dosing, follow the package labeling accurately.

HOMEOPATHIC REMEDIES (For quick reference please refer to the "Homeopathic Remedies List" on page 32 and the inside cover.)

- A homeopathic cream designed to soothe inflamed or irritated skin may be useful. It may also promote skin healing. It can be applied directly to the affected area 3 times a day. (Skin 1)

BACH FLOWER REMEDIES

- Rescue Remedy™ may be of use if your child is uncomfortable from the illness, stress, or anxiety. You may use 2 drops every 10 minutes to every few hours to calm restlessness as needed.

NUTRITIONALS AND SUPPLEMENTS

- Vitamin A
- Vitamin E
- EFAs
- Probiotics

 When to Call Your Health-care Provider

Call immediately if any of the following occur:

- Your child's urine becomes red- or brown-colored.
- Your child's face becomes very swollen, bright red, and tender to the touch.
- Your child is so uncomfortable that he cannot be consoled.

Call within 24 hours if:

- Any big blisters (more than $1/2$ inch across) develop.
- The impetigo increases in size and number of sores, even after 48 hours of treatment.
- A fever (greater than 104 degrees) occurs.
- Your child complains of a sore throat.
- A red area develops, spreading away from the impetigo.

IMPETIGO

 Other Relevant Sections

Chickenpox

Hives

 Prevention

Impetigo can be spread by direct contact. When your child touches the impetigo and then scratches another part of the skin, a new site of impetigo may develop. To prevent this spread, encourage your child not to touch, scratch, or pick these sores. Encourage your child to keep his fingers out of his nose. Teach your child good hand-washing techniques. Keep fingernails cut short, and clean your child's hands and nails thoroughly with antibacterial soap.

Children with impetigo should be isolated, as much as possible, from others until 24 hours after antibiotics have been started. Do not allow your own child to play with any child with impetigo who has not been properly treated.

If another child in the family develops the same lesions and at least one child has been seen by your health-care provider to establish the correct diagnosis, your health-care provider may consider a prescription over the phone for a second child.

"MONO"

 ### Description/Physiology

Infectious mononucleosis, commonly called "mono," is a viral illness that affects children of a variety of ages, particularly adolescents. It is often referred to as the "kissing disease" because adolescents may pass it from one partner to another by kissing, though kissing is not required for transmission.

Mono can be a very benign illness with minimal symptoms, a moderately severe illness with some debilitation and discomfort, or a severe illness with incapacitating symptoms and significant loss of school days and regular activity. It is often mistaken for influenza or the "flu" in its early stages.

The mono virus attacks the body's immune system and infects the throat, lymph nodes (glands), liver, and spleen. A sore throat is the primary feature. The sore throat is often accompanied by swollen lymph nodes in the neck, armpits, and/or groin, which not only are enlarged but often quite tender. In the early stages of the disease, there may be a fever that ranges from 100 to 104 degrees. Fever may last up to 7 to 14 days. Exhaustion is another hallmark of mono. Children will sleep for very long stretches of time and may show little or no interest in exercise or eating.

Mono is diagnosed by a blood test, either a "monospot," which gives us an answer within several hours, or the more accurate Epstein-Barr virus (EBV) titers, which take a few days to be measured. Both of these tests are done in a laboratory.

 ### Causes/Epidemiology

Infectious mononucleosis (mono) is caused by the Epstein-Barr virus (EBV). This virus is transmitted through oral and nasal secretions and is easily transmitted to a new host. The incubation period is roughly 30 to 50 days after exposure. In addition, a "mono-like syndrome" can be produced by a number of different viruses. These viruses create symptoms that can appear exactly like mono, but your child will not test positive for mono. The mono virus can be shed up to 6 months after the infection.

Expected Course

Most young children with mono have only mild symptoms lasting less than 1 week. Thus, some cases of mono may pass undiagnosed because the symptoms will often disappear before there is a need for medical evaluation. There may be a loss of normal appetite, a bit more sleeping than usual, and some generalized achiness. These children may feel well enough to attend school and are often thought to simply have a "flu bug."

Other children, especially adolescents, can be significantly debilitated by mono. They present with very sore throats, high fevers, markedly enlarged lymph nodes (especially in the head and neck regions), abdominal pain, headache, malaise, dramatically increased sleep requirements, a red rash, chills, and generalized muscle aches. Even adolescents with these prolonged and more extreme symptoms may feel better within 2 to 4 weeks.

The most severe mono cases may keep a child out of school for several days and even weeks. Symptoms may improve only very slowly, and it may be a month or two for full recovery to take place. Some adolescents report that they do not feel completely back to normal for as many as 6 months!

Complications of mono are rare, and the most common acute complication is dehydration triggered by painful swallowing and decreased fluid intake. The throat may be sore enough that a child will refuse fluids altogether. This may require an ER visit and IV hydration. Some children are so uncomfortable, dehydrated, and/or have significant breathing disruption that hospitalization is required.

A child's breathing may be compromised because of enlarged tonsils and may result in restless sleep and agitation. The back of the throat may become so swollen that harsh breathing and snoring may be present.

Your child may feel discomfort of the abdomen just below the rib cage because the liver can also be involved; some children develop a form of viral hepatitis from the mono virus that may cause abdominal pain and even jaundice. The spleen may also be abnormally large, and rarely, an injury to the abdomen (in the left upper quadrant) may cause a rupture of the spleen and thus a surgical emergency. See below.

Depending on the length of the illness and your child's emotional state, anxiety and depression may develop. These children are exhausted by the illness, its severity, its length, their slow recovery, the loss of normal activity, weight loss, and loss of contact with peers and the school environment. Many children may be worried about lost school days and the possibility of failing grades.

Since mono and strep may occur simultaneously, children with mono who have persistent and worsening sore throats should be evaluated with an examination and a strep test.

 ## Contagiousness/Immunity

Infectious mononucleosis is contagious. As mentioned, the virus is transmitted in oral and nasal secretions. The virus can be passed on contaminated hands, on contaminated objects (such as toys—the virus may survive for several hours on inanimate objects), through kissing, sharing saliva-contaminated utensils, water bottles and glasses, and even on towels and pillowcases. Mono is not easily passed through the air, but a cough or sneeze can transmit the virus, as well.

Meticulous hand-washing and reasonable efforts at isolation of your child and his secretions will reduce the potential for spread. It is difficult to pinpoint exactly when a child is no longer contagious, but he is likely most contagious during the fever phase.

In general, a child only suffers from mono once in his life.

 ## Home Care

Mono is a viral infection, so there is no specific treatment that cures mono. The goals are to provide comfort and relief for the most distressing symptoms and to support your child through his own natural healing process. In addition, you must remain vigilant for complications of mono.

We ask you to first read through the entire "Home Care" section and select those recommendations that make the most sense for your child's current situation.

1. Aches and pain relief. Symptoms such as the pain of swollen lymph nodes, sore throat, and general body aches can usually be relieved by acetaminophen or ibuprofen. See "OTC Medication Recommendations and Dosages" section. Ibuprofen is the preferred preparation. We never recommend the use of aspirin during a mono illness.

2. Sore throat treatment. See "Throat" section. Older children may gargle with warm salt water ($1/2$ teaspoon of salt per glass) or an antacid solution, such as Maalox®. Sucking on hard candy may also relieve sore throat symptoms. Butterscotch seems to be a particularly soothing flavor.

3. Diet. Since swollen, inflamed tonsils may make some foods difficult to swallow, provide a soft diet. Dairy products may produce additional mucous, so avoid them unless that is all your child will eat. Bland, easy-to-digest foods are best.

4. Hydration. To prevent dehydration, be sure that your child drinks sufficient fluids. See "Dehydration" section. Sore throat pain may dramatically reduce fluid intake, and coupled with the evaporative losses of fluid from the fever, may cause dehydration. Frequent, small sips of soothing clear liquids, fruit juices, popsicles, and clear soup broths are best.

5. Activity. Your child does not absolutely need to stay in bed at all times. He may select how much rest he needs. Usually, children will voluntarily "slow down" until the fever and major symptoms have resolved. After a few days like this, however, your child will be restless, so be prepared with some "effort-free" measures that provide good distractions, such as movies, books, and games. Most children will return to full activity within 2 to 4 weeks as long as there are no further complications.

6. Precautions for an enlarged spleen. A small percentage of children with mono will have an enlarged spleen that can no longer be protected from trauma by the rib cage. Once your health-care provider has confirmed an enlarged spleen by direct exam, it is important to protect the abdomen from injury (especially from contact sports). Thus, children with an enlarged spleen should be restricted from high-risk activities until declared medically safe. It is prudent that all children with mono avoid contact sports for at least four weeks or longer, as directed by your health-care provider.

 ## Integrated Therapies

(Please refer to the section on "Administering Integrated Treatments" on page 19 for guidance on using any of the therapies that follow.)

AROMATHERAPY

- An aromatherapy bath or massage with the essential oils of eucalyptus radiata and/or lavender can soothe and relax your child's anxiety and restlessness as well as his congestion and difficult breathing. Add 2 to 5 drops of oil to a warm bath and allow your child to soak for a comfortable period of time.

HERBAL REMEDIES (For quick reference please refer to the "Herbal Remedies List" on page 31 and the inside cover.)

- Echinacea can be used to support the immune system in helping to resolve a viral infection. For dosing, follow the package labeling accurately.
- Valerian root is a mild herbal sedative that may offer some help in easing a child with significant restlessness or pain. Valerian root may be most useful at bedtime. For dosing, follow the package labeling accurately.

HOMEOPATHIC REMEDIES (For quick reference please refer to the "Homeopathic Remedies List" on page 32 and the inside cover.)

- A homeopathic remedy designed to support the defense systems in viral infections may be useful. It can be taken 3 to 6 times daily when the virus is active (for example, fever, lethargy, etc.). (General Support 1)
- A homeopathic remedy designed to relieve some of the discomforts associated with infections (for example, fever, body aches, chills, and fatigue) may be useful. It can be taken 3 to 6 times daily when the virus is active (for example, fever, lethargy, etc.). (General Support 3)
- A homeopathic remedy designed to relieve acute and severe inflammation may be helpful when given for severe sore throat pain or swollen, tender lymph nodes. It may be taken 3 times daily for up to 3 days. If no relief is achieved within 3 days, you should consult your health-care provider. (General Support 5)
- A homeopathic remedy designed to help reduce the impact of the fatigue that can be associated with mono may be helpful. It may be taken 3 times daily for as long as there is fatigue. (General Support 6)
- A homeopathic remedy designed to minimize dizziness, which can be a frustrating symptom of mono, may help to relieve it. It may be taken 3 times daily for as long as there is dizziness. (General Support 7)

BACH FLOWER REMEDIES

- Rescue Remedy™ may be of use if your child is uncomfortable from the illness, stress, or anxiety. You may use 2 drops every 10 minutes to every few hours to calm restlessness as needed.
- A lukewarm bath with 10 drops of Rescue Remedy™ added to the bathwater is often very effective at relieving agitation and stress in general.
- Olive remedy, by Bach Flower™, can be very helpful to alleviate both mental and physical fatigue. It can be administered as 2 drops directly in the mouth 1 to 2 times a day for as long as there is fatigue.

NUTRITIONALS AND SUPPLEMENTS

- Vitamin C
- A good multivitamin and multi-mineral supplement may be very beneficial to prevent or minimize the protracted nature of mono
- Zinc
- EFAs

DIETARY GUIDELINES

- Reduce or eliminate fried and fatty foods and sugar-sweetened foods from the diet.
- Eliminate alcohol and caffeine intake.
- Warm foods such as soups, warm cooked grains (for example, oatmeal), and teas should be given.
- It is best to avoid all dairy products and citrus fruits because they may increase or thicken respiratory mucous.
- Your child may not feel well enough to eat, so don't force food. Instead, make sure that he continues a good intake of fluids and drinks extra water to ensure good hydration. You may use the following table as a general guideline for water in addition to normal fluid intake:

AGE	OUNCES OF WATER PER DAY
2 to 5 years old	12 to 18 ounces
5 to 12 years old	18 to 24 ounces
13 and up	32 to 48 ounces

INTEGRATIVE SUPPORTIVE CARE

- Please read the section "Integrated Management of Respiratory Illnesses."

 When to Call Your Health-care Provider

Call immediately if any of the following occur:
- Breathing becomes difficult or labored.
- Your child becomes so agitated or anxious that he cannot be easily consoled or calmed.
- Significant abdominal pain develops.
- Bleeding into the skin occurs, creating heavily bruised areas.
- Your child has not urinated in the last 12 hours. See "Dehydration" section.
- Your child's temperature exceeds 105 degrees. See "Fever" section.

Call within 24 hours if:
- Your child becomes dehydrated.
- Swallowing becomes increasingly difficult.
- Sleeping becomes increasingly disrupted.

- Sinus or ear pain develops.
- Your child's fever is still present after 10 days.
- Your child isn't back to school within 2 weeks.
- Your child develops jaundiced or yellow skin.

 ## Other Relevant Sections

Abdominal Pain

Dehydration

Fever

Headaches

Influenza

Lymph Nodes

Throat

Integrated Management of Respiratory Illnesses

 ## Prevention

Prevention of mono is often difficult because contact with infected secretions can happen without our knowledge. Your child can be exposed to mono at school or daycare.

Prevention of mono requires careful attention to guarding against the spread of contaminated oral and nasal secretions. Careful hand-washing is the cornerstone of prevention. You should wash your own hands carefully anytime you come into direct contact with your ill child or any objects he may have handled. This is especially true for cups and eating utensils. Remind your child not to share water bottles or drinks with others, even if they seem healthy.

It is best to keep your child away from any child with known mono at least until the fever has disappeared and the other generalized symptoms have begun to resolve. Your healthy child should be encouraged not to share cups, food, utensils, or handle any objects touched by the infected child, or any child for that matter.

Description/Physiology

Influenza ("the flu") is a viral infection that affects the nose, throat, and lungs. It occurs every year, primarily in December through March. The main symptoms are stuffy nose, sore throat, cough, fatigue, headache, and muscle aches. For most children, influenza is very much like a typical viral infection.

Causes/Epidemiology

Influenza is caused by the influenza virus. In any given year, there are approximately 3 or 4 main influenza viral strains that account for the majority of the influenza that we see. In addition, a dozen or more viruses can cause "influenza-like" symptoms. This is why we often refer to it as the "flu," because it is difficult to know for certain if the virus is influenza or another virus, although influenza usually causes a more miserable illness. Because all of these virus groups cause similar symptoms and the treatment for all of them is the same, we will discuss them as if they were a single disease—"the flu."

These viruses enter the body through the respiratory tract, primarily the nose or mouth, and immediately invade these membranes. These tissues become inflamed and swollen, and then mucous is produced. The virus easily enters the bloodstream and can be circulated throughout the rest of the body. That is why we often hear, "My whole body aches!"

Significant influenza epidemics occur every 2 or 3 years, with milder versions in between. There is never a year that passes without an "influenza season."

Expected Course

Children respond to the flu in a variety of ways. In infants, the illness can be severe, since babies have difficulty localizing the infection to one location, such as the throat. These children can be restless, eat and drink less, and have significant fever and lethargy.

Older children and adolescents may have very mild symptoms much like a cold, with low-grade fever (100 to 102 degrees), a dry and hacking cough, headache, and muscle aches. With minimal treatment they are often better within just a few days.

Some children may have a more severe syndrome. They may have a much higher fever (102 to 106 degrees), extreme irritability when awake, increased lethargy, a very sore throat, a painful and unremitting cough, decreased appetite, sleep disruption, and severe muscle aches. These children may be bedridden for up to a week before some activity is resumed. Even then, it may take an additional week or two for full recovery to take place.

In the most severe cases, some children will require evaluation beyond your health-care provider and a visit to the ER for further diagnostic evaluation and possibly IV fluids. Hospitalization is less likely. Children with severe flu may experience complications such as pneumonia, bronchitis, and dehydration, although these are rare.

Healthy children less than 2 years of age and children with underlying health problems, such as asthma and diabetes, are especially prone to more severe versions of the flu. For these children an influenza vaccine each year is highly recommended.

Contagiousness/Immunity

Influenza is highly contagious. It is transmitted in the air by a cough or sneeze. It is also passed along in infected secretions from an ill child. It enters the respiratory tract through the nose, mouth, and/or eye.

Because there are so many different strains of virus that can cause the flu, it is possible to have a flu syndrome more than once in a single season. Having one episode of "the flu" confers no protection against another "flu-like" virus.

Your child is contagious about 2 days before the onset of symptoms and will continue to be contagious at least until the fever is gone and other symptoms begin to resolve. It is impossible to know exactly when the virus has made its final exit from your child's body; however, your child can generally return to school or daycare when the fever is gone for at least 24 hours and symptoms are mild enough to resume normal activity.

Home Care

The treatment of influenza depends on your child's age, severity of symptoms, and any other underlying illnesses your child may have. Our goals are to provide comfort and to support your child's own immune system to fight the infection. Treatment is similar to that for other viral respiratory infections.

We ask you to first read through the entire "Home Care" section to select the recommendations that make the most sense for your child's current situation.

1. Fever. Use acetaminophen or ibuprofen. See "OTC Medication Recommendations and Dosages" section. When your child has a fever but is comfortable, it is fine to watch him carefully without administering

these medications, to allow the body's own natural healing mechanism to attack the virus. If the presence of the fever causes your child any pain or discomfort, he should be treated with pain-relieving medication (acetaminophen or ibuprofen). See "Fever" section for further guidance on fever management.

Aspirin should be avoided in all children and adolescents with suspected influenza.

2. Aches. Muscle aches, especially in older children, can be very debilitating. Here again, ibuprofen or acetaminophen can help. Gentle massage may also relieve some muscle tightness and provide relief.

3. Cough. See "Cough" section. The primary goal is to provide relief so that your child can sleep. This may require the use of a cough suppressant. During the day, we discourage cough suppressants so that mucous can be mobilized and coughed out of the respiratory tract. Elevating the head of the bed and running a vaporizer during sleep are helpful relief measures for the cough. Should your child need a cough suppressant in order to sleep, see "OTC Medication Recommendations and Dosages" section.

4. Sore throat. See "Throat" section for a more complete discussion.

5. Congestion. Use saline nose drops made of $1/2$ teaspoon of salt and 1 cup of water or commercially available saline drops (for example, Ocean®). Put 2 drops in each nostril and have your child blow his nose or you may suction away the mucous. Repeat as needed 3 to 4 times per day.

If nasal congestion significantly interferes with eating or sleeping and saline nose drops are not sufficient, you may consider using OTC phenylephrine nose drops in a strength of $1/8$% or $1/4$%. You may administer 1 to 2 drops in each nostril as needed to support eating and sleeping for a maximum of 3 doses per day, for a maximum of 7 days. (Use for longer periods can result in nasal membrane dependency.) Either cool-mist or warm-mist humidifiers or vaporizers can be helpful.

6. Hydration. We recommend ample clear liquids to maintain hydration and thin the mucous so that it can be expelled more easily from the respiratory tract. Milk and other dairy products tend to produce mucous, which further worsens the situation. Popsicles, $1/2$ strength Gatorade®, soups, diluted juices, and warm teas are soothing. These fluids may also help with constipation caused by decreased oral intake. See "Dehydration" section.

7. Nutrition. A diet of soft foods, easy to digest and low in fat is best. Fruits, cereal, and bland solids are fine.

8. Eliminate cigarette smoke.

Integrated Therapies

(Please refer to the section on "Administering Integrated Treatments" on page 19 for guidance on using any of the therapies that follow.)

AROMATHERAPY

- Ravensara aromatica essential oil may have a preventive effect for influenza when a child has a significant exposure or when used early in the illness. Add 2 to 5 drops of oil to a warm bath and allow your child to soak for a comfortable period of time. You may also add 2 to 3 drops to a tablespoon of olive oil and rub into the bottoms of the feet, the chest, and back. It may also be used as a steam inhalation.
- An aromatherapy bath or massage with the essential oils of eucalyptus radiata and/or lavender can soothe and relax your child's anxiety and restlessness. Add 2 to 3 drops of oil to a warm bath and allow your child to soak for a comfortable period of time.

HERBAL REMEDIES (For quick reference please refer to the "Herbal Remedies List" on page 31 and the inside cover.)

- Echinacea can be used to support the immune system in helping to resolve a viral infection. For dosing, follow the package labeling accurately.
- Horehound may be very effective in reducing mucous production and thus improve a wet cough. It may help in the recuperative phase of bronchitis, if there is a significant amount of mucous production. For dosing, follow the package labeling accurately.
- Valerian root is a mild herbal sedative that may offer some help in easing a child with significant restlessness. Valerian root may be most useful at bedtime. For dosing, follow the package labeling accurately.
- Herbal teas may offer some soothing relief of cold symptoms (especially a sore throat) and also provide a good source of fluids. Herb teas made from chamomile or mint as well as a variety of blended herbal teas can be brewed according to package directions, sweetened to taste, and offered frequently throughout the day.

HOMEOPATHIC REMEDIES (For quick reference please refer to the "Homeopathic Remedies List" on page 32 and the inside cover.)

- A homeopathic remedy designed to support the defense system in viral infections may be useful. It can be taken 3 to 6 times daily when the virus is active (for example, fever, lethargy, etc.). (General Support 1)

229

- A homeopathic remedy designed to relieve some of the discomforts associated with infections (for example, fever, body aches, chills and fatigue) may be useful. It can be taken 3 to 6 times daily when the virus is active (for example, fever, lethargy, etc.). (General Support 3)
- A homeopathic remedy designed to minimize nasal congestion and mucous, especially when associated with respiratory infections, may be useful. It can be taken 2 to 3 times daily while there is nasal congestion. (Respiratory 3)

BACH FLOWER REMEDIES

- Rescue Remedy™ may be of use if your child is uncomfortable from the illness, stress, or anxiety. You may use 2 drops every 10 minutes to every few hours to calm restlessness as needed.
- Ten drops of Rescue Remedy™ added to a lukewarm bath is often very effective at relieving many of the symptoms of the flu.

NUTRITIONALS AND SUPPLEMENTS

- Vitamin A
- Vitamin C
- Zinc

DIETARY GUIDELINES

- It is best to avoid all dairy products and citrus fruits because they may increase or thicken respiratory mucous.
- Reduce or eliminate fried and fatty foods and sugar-sweetened foods from the diet.
- Eliminate alcohol and caffeine intake.
- Warm foods such as soups, warm cooked grains (for example, oatmeal), and teas should be given.
- Your child may not feel well enough to eat, so don't force food. Instead, make sure that he continues a good intake of fluids and drinks extra water to ensure good hydration. You may use the following table as a general guideline for water in addition to normal fluid intake:

AGE	OUNCES OF WATER PER DAY
2 to 5 years old	12 to 18 ounces
5 to 12 years old	18 to 24 ounces
13 and up	32 to 48 ounces

INTEGRATIVE SUPPORTIVE CARE

- Please read the section "Integrated Management of Respiratory Illnesses."

 When to Call Your Health-care Provider

Call immediately if any of the following occur:

- Your child becomes progressively restless or agitated in spite of adequate pain management.
- Your child becomes progressively more lethargic and difficult to arouse.
- Your child complains of a stiff neck, blurred vision, or cannot walk.
- Your child exhibits signs of dehydration. See "Dehydration" section.
- Your child coughs up blood.
- Your child develops a fever greater than 106 degrees. See "Fever" section.
- Your child complains of severe chest or abdominal pain not relieved within an hour.
- Shortness of breath or rapid breathing rate (over 60 breaths per minute in an infant or over 40 breaths per minute in children over the age of 2 years), especially in the absence of fever.
- Your young child or infant has significant difficulty breathing and/or croup-like stridor when taking a breath. See "Croup" section.

Call within 24 hours if:

- An earache develops.
- Fever lasts more than four days.
- Difficulty with breathing is gradually worsening.
- Your child has not been able to return to school for over a week.
- Your child has a severe sore throat and has been exposed to strep.

 Other Relevant Sections

Bronchitis
Colds
Cough

231

Croup

Dehydration

Earache/Ear Infection

Infectious Mononucleosis

Throat

Integrated Management of Respiratory Illnesses

 Prevention

Influenza viruses are transmitted through the air and through oral and nasal secretions. It is impossible to prevent every contact, especially in public places. Hand-washing is the key to spreading the virus. Caregivers and parents should wash their hands thoroughly after handling a sick child and/or objects touched by that child. The virus may survive on inanimate surfaces for several hours and so can be passed along on contaminated toys, books, and clothing.

It is also important to teach your children to wash their hands regularly as well as to cover their nose and mouth when sneezing and coughing. Avoid children who are known to be ill. This is especially true if your child is prone to infections.

If your child is prone to emotional stress, seek out factors in his environment that act as triggers for illness and work to lessen or minimize them.

Finally, an influenza vaccine, or the "flu shot," is available. This shot is available in the fall every year and is specific for only the influenza virus. It does not protect against any of the other viruses that cause "flu-like" illnesses. All children, 6 months to 23 months of age, and children with underlying issues (asthma, premature infants, children on oxygen, diabetics, cystic fibrosis, etc.) are encouraged to receive the flu vaccine yearly. In otherwise normal children, the influenza vaccine is optional and a parental choice. The "flu shot" is a "killed virus" vaccine, and therefore cannot give your child the flu. Rarely, the "flu shot" may cause a mild "flu-like" reaction or low-grade fever for 1 to 2 days following the injection.

This section is designed to cover many of the care aspects common to respiratory illnesses, without having to repeat it at the end of every respiratory illness section throughout our handbook. Paying close attention to the details of care in this section is as important to enhancing your child's recovery as are the details found in the specific illness section.

ENVIRONMENT: Your child should be kept in the same familiar surroundings of his own home and bedroom whenever possible. To relax and be comfortable enough to rest in a less familiar place is difficult for most children, and valuable energy is lost in trying to do so.

Most activities, especially physical activities, should be limited, although children who are mildly ill often enjoy a quiet board game or reading. Children who are more miserable might prefer the distractions of watching TV and videos or listening to music. Phone calls and visitors should be restricted so that your child can really rest. It is preferable that children do not leave home at all, or only for absolutely essential needs such as a visit to the doctor or the pharmacy, as trips away from home can be particularly stressful to ill children.

Consider silencing the phone for part of the day. Lie down yourself and rest to make up for the deficit in rest that you, as the caregiver, have undoubtedly experienced from lost sleep and the hard work of supporting your child through this illness.

A lukewarm bath can be very comforting to an ill child, especially with the added essential oils (bath and massage oil) of eucalyptus radiata and/or lavender. Make sure the water temperature is not too cool, to avoid creating a chill which could further increase your child's discomfort. Even if your child has a fever, warm bathwater is cooler than the feverish child and thus will not increase the fever. Instead, the warm water will often soothe aching muscles and help your child relax.

A gentle massage is another wonderful way to soothe and relax your child. This not only eases restlessness, it also gives him the added therapeutic benefit of your physical touch. Even if you don't know a specific massage technique, your loving, gentle touch will make your child feel cared for in a way for which there is no substitute.

You can keep children from either chilling or overheating by dressing them in layers. The appropriate amount of clothing is that which keeps the child comfortable enough to rest. Some children prefer more layers and some prefer less. Follow your child's lead and your own instincts. If your child has a fever, you may want to dress him lightly so the heat can dissipate more readily. Regardless of fever, however, if your child is chilled, you should keep him dressed more warmly.

Even indoors, an ill child may need a hat and socks or slippers to stay warm, because much heat can be lost through a child's head and feet.

It is very important to pay close attention to the air your child breathes while he has a respiratory illness. There should be absolutely no exposure to any cigarette smoke, paint or other vapors, or dust (from vacuuming, sanding of wood, etc.). Any known allergens, for example, cat or dog dander, should be minimized or avoided. Humidification of the air is not only soothing but also promotes healing. While steam vaporizers provide the cleanest source of humidification, they also pose a risk of burning an unattended child. Cool-mist humidifiers must be cleaned at least weekly (according to the manufacturer's specifications) to avoid mold buildup. They pose no risk of burning a child.

Using an air purifier in your child's room can help prevent and/or resolve respiratory illnesses. A good room air purifier can remove 99 percent of pollutants, allergens, dust, animal dander, and "germs" from the air. This air purification could benefit any child with a respiratory illness, but is especially helpful for children with chronic respiratory illnesses.

Air purifiers generally use HEPA filter technology, which is an excellent method. Most department stores, hardware stores, and pharmacies carry affordable room air purifiers with this HEPA technology.

Elevating your child's head will help improve the comfort associated with the natural drainage of mucous during a respiratory infection. For older children, prop them up on pillows or have them relax in a reclining chair. Infants and toddlers are often very comfortable in their car seat, which can be placed in their crib or on the floor. This elevates their head and they are often able to sleep very comfortably for naps and bedtime.

PAIN RELIEF: When children have respiratory illnesses, especially those caused by infections, they may suffer from several simultaneous complaints such as earache, headache, sore throat, and general muscle aches. Younger children may not be able to communicate their specific complaints; therefore, their pain might manifest as restlessness, irritability, or lethargy.

Some children, in spite of mild discomforts, may be able to sleep on and off all day long and thus have no need for specific intervention for their pain. However, many children are uncomfortable enough that they will need medications for pain relief. Acetaminophen and ibuprofen are the safest and most effective pain relievers for children. (Please refer to the "OTC Medication Recommendations and Dosages" section.)

Sore throat pain can be most difficult to relieve, but along with the pain relievers listed above, you may give your older child throat lozenges (for example, Original Ricola® Herbal Cough Drops). There are also a variety of herbal teas that soothe throat pain when sipped (for example, Throat Coat® Tea by Traditional Medicinals). OTC throat sprays such as Chloraseptic® or Sore Throat Spray™ by Herbs for Kids may also provide some relief. (For dosing, follow package directions accurately.)

Oftentimes when your child has taken pain-relieving medication, he will appear to have almost miraculously improved. While you will be grateful for the respite from the misery, you should be careful not to be fooled by it. This should be your opportunity to encourage more rest, not more activity, even if your child is trying to talk you into a concession—for example, having a friend over or playing in the park.

If these medications, along with specific measures found elsewhere in this handbook, do not adequately relieve your child's pain and discomfort, please call your health-care provider to discuss it further.

SLEEP: Most children who are ill will want to sleep more if they are not in pain and are not uncomfortable. Pain relievers will usually relieve discomfort enough that, if they want to fall asleep, they will. However, in spite of the pain-relief measures listed above, on occasion a child will still be too restless to get to sleep. In such cases valerian root is a safe and usually effective method to help restless children fall asleep. Please refer to the "Herbal Therapies" section for further guidance. For dosing, follow the package guidelines accurately. Rescue Remedy™ may also be of use if your child is agitated or restless. You may use 2 drops every 10 to 60 minutes to calm restlessness, as needed. In cases where the child is still unable to fall asleep, your health-care provider may occasionally prescribe a sedative.

Children generally sleep best in their own beds or with you in your bed. Don't be afraid of lying down or sleeping with your child, as this rarely leads to habit formation. Even if it does, the short-lived habit can be dealt with relatively easily once he is well. The only real risk of lying down with your child is his contagiousness to you. Only you can assess how much exposure risk you are willing to take. The extra rest that you all may get could be more valuable in the long run.

RUNNY NOSE AND NASAL CONGESTION: With most respiratory illnesses there is a component of a runny nose and/or nasal congestion (stuffiness). Many OTC preparations contain decongestants and/or antihistamines for relief of the runny nose and congestion. We feel strongly, however, that oral antihistamines and decongestants should be avoided. While they may offer minimal relief, it is

INTEGRATED MANAGEMENT OF RESPIRATORY ILLNESSES

generally short-lived. They may also have some significant side effects. They may cause restlessness and agitation in some children. In our opinion, these preparations can also thicken the mucous in the nose, middle ear, and sinuses and this can significantly diminish the ability of the mucous to drain. The lack of drainage increases the risk of mucous trapping and becoming secondarily infected with bacteria (that is, sinus or ear infections).

If you feel that some treatment is required, you may begin with salt water (saline) nasal irrigation. In small children, first clear the nostrils with a bulb syringe and then use nose drops (saline) made of $1/2$ teaspoon of salt and 1 cup of water or you may use OTC preparations such as Ocean®. Put 2 drops in each nostril, and suction out the mucous. Repeat as needed 3 to 4 times per day, but remember that nasal suctioning too frequently can cause the nasal membrane to swell, which worsens congestion.

If a child's congestion or nasal drainage is significant enough to affect his ability to eat, sleep, or rest comfortably, a nasal spray decongestant may be used. Please refer to the "OTC Medication Recommendations and Dosages" section for further guidance. For dosing, follow the package guidelines accurately. These medications also run the risk of causing a "rebound" effect if they are used for a prolonged period of time. A rebound effect means that, after the medication has worn off, the symptoms return to a level of severity worse than the original level. Rebounds are uncommon if the product is used only 2 to 3 times per day for less than 5 days.

Another useful approach involves using a homeopathic nose spray remedy. Please refer to the remedy listed as Respiratory 3 on "The Homeopathic Remedies List." This nasal spray is designed to keep the nasal membranes from swelling and to minimize the amount of mucous produced. It can be given in a dose of 1 spray in each nostril 2 to 3 times daily. While it can be used in conjunction with the OTC nasal spray decongestants, they should be given at least 1 hour apart. This remedy is also available as an oral remedy and may be given 2 to 3 times daily, as well.

COUGH: Cough is one of the most disruptive and uncomfortable symptoms of a respiratory illness. It is so important that an entire chapter has been dedicated to its management. Please refer to the "Cough" section in this book, as it covers all aspects of cough.

DIET: Children generally lose their appetite when they are ill, and you should follow their lead carefully. If they are not hungry, do not force them to eat, and especially do not offer them junk food alternatives just to bribe them to eat. If

236

they are hungry, feed them simple foods, preferably well-cooked, such as cooked grains (rice, oatmeal, pasta) and cooked vegetables or fruit (canned peaches). It is far more important that an ill child drink plenty of fluids than eat solid foods.

SUPPLEMENTS:

Vitamin C:

The use of Vitamin C to prevent respiratory infections and minimize respiratory symptoms is still controversial. We do recommend the use of Vitamin C in safe doses. Our experience suggests that some children clearly benefit, while others do not. Therefore, you must judge for yourself the impact of vitamin C on your own child's health. The vitamin C doses that we recommend during a cold are as follows:

12 months to 2 years	100 mg 3-4 times daily
2 years to 5 years	250 mg 3-4 times daily
5 years to 10 years	500 mg 3-4 times daily
10 years and up	1,000 mg 3-4 times daily

Zinc:

Zinc is one of the most important nutrients supporting the function of the immune system and as such, zinc supplementation may benefit the immune response at the onset of a respiratory infection. Zinc may also possess a topical inhibitory effect on an invading virus, thus enhancing the body's ability to help fend off respiratory infections. Zinc comes in a variety of products, including a homeopathic form, and is safe for use in children when used in strict accordance with the dosing and administration guidelines found on the product package.

Zinc also comes in the form of a lollypop or sucker on a stick (for example, Zinc Pops), which is suitable for children 6 months or older. Again, follow the dosing guidelines on the package insert.

There are also numerous brands of zinc lozenges (and suckers for younger children) suitable for anyone old enough to safely suck a hard candy. It is recommended that you follow the dosing guidelines on the product you are using. NOTE: Many of these products contain other herbs (for example, echinacea) and nutrient supplements (for example, vitamin C). These ingredients should be considered part of the total daily dose of those particular supplements, to avoid the risk of overdose.

Zinc is most effective when taken as early in the illness as possible and then

INTEGRATED MANAGEMENT OF RESPIRATORY ILLNESSES

continued for 2 to 5 days. However, zinc supplementation should not be used for more than 7 days, as it can lose its effectiveness and there is a greater chance for intolerance with prolonged use. For dosing zinc suckers and lozenges, always follow the package guidelines. If there are no guidelines, you may safely follow the guidelines below.

AGE	MAXIMUM DAILY DOSE
	(for a maximum of 7 days)
6 to 12 months	6 mg
1 to 2 years	10 mg
3 to 12 years	10 mg
12 years and up	15 mg

Vitamin A:

Vitamin A is essential to the immune system since it is required for and can stimulate multiple functions in the immune system. It is also a critical nutrient for the repair and maintenance of the cells of mucosal surfaces (that is, the surfaces that line the entire respiratory tract). These two aspects of vitamin A make it an important nutrient to use as a supplement to support children with respiratory illnesses, especially infections. Vitamin A may be given once daily for 1 to 2 weeks using the following dosing guidelines:

AGE	MAXIMUM DAILY DOSE
	GIVEN ONCE A DAY
1 to 3 years	2,000 IU
4 to 6 years	2,500 IU
7 to 10 years	3,500 IU
11 years and up	4,000 IU

Echinacea/astragalus:

Echinacea/astragalus is a combination herbal remedy that may have a significant effect on enhancing the immune system's response to a developing infection. It is available in many forms (tea, capsules, and tinctures), but is most effective if given in the tincture form and as early in the illness as possible. It may be given 3 to 5 times per day for the first 2 to 3 days and then 2 to 3 times a day for 1 to 2 days more. Please refer to the "Herbal Remedies List."

Echinacea/astragalus may also help children resist colds and flu when used regularly throughout the winter months. Please consult your health-care provider for further information. Because echinacea/astragalus can stimulate the immune system, it should not be used in diseases where the immune system is already overactive—for example, asthma and eczema. If your child

238

develops a rash, wheezing, or other allergic symptoms while taking echinacea/astragalus, you should discontinue its use and contact your health-care provider for advice.

"SWOLLEN GLANDS"

 Description/Physiology

Normal-sized lymph nodes are generally less than $1/2$ inch in diameter, roughly the size of a pea. There are several hundred superficial lymph nodes we can feel under the skin. There are more than 100 lymph nodes in the head and neck region alone. The groin and armpits are other sites with a large concentration of lymph nodes.

Lymph nodes are part of the body's immune system. They are sentinels that protect a particular region of the body. They drain and eliminate toxins from the surface of the body (for example, bug bites and splinters). They help protect the bloodstream from invasion by both viruses and bacteria, which prevents or stops the spread of infection. We see this in the child who has a cold virus, which produces a sore throat, nasal congestion, and fever. The lymph nodes in these areas drain toxins, the inflammatory cell debris, and infectious materials away from the site of infection, and serve as temporary storage sites for this immune debris.

When a child develops a viral or bacterial infection, lymph nodes in that area are activated for protection. They drain the germs and dead cell debris and provide protective white blood cells and other immune support factors to halt the spread of infection into deeper tissues. Activated lymph nodes are often mildly tender and swollen, though usually no more than $1/2$ to 1 inch in diameter.

If the virus or bacteria overwhelm the lymph node itself, lymph nodes will usually be more than 1 inch in diameter and may be externally tender to the touch. This may be the beginning of a bacterial infection in the lymph node itself. Signs that the nodes may be infected are that the glands are over 1 inch in diameter; the skin overlaying the gland is pink or red; and/or they are very tender.

 Causes/Epidemiology

In addition to the invading viruses and bacteria, lymph nodes can be swollen because of skin damaged by cuts, scrapes, scratches, splinters, burns, insect bites, rashes, impetigo, or any disruption in the normal skin barrier. Altogether, these sources probably account for 98 percent of all swollen lymph nodes, with viruses playing a role in 75 percent of cases.

To locate and identify the source of the inflammation that causes a swollen gland, some simple principles of anatomy may help. The nodes of the groin area drain the legs and lower abdomen; the armpit nodes drain the arms and upper chest; the back-of-the-neck nodes drain the scalp; and the front-of-the-neck nodes drain the face, nose, and throat.

Most enlarged head and neck nodes are due to colds. With the usual viral infections, bacterial infections, or skin injuries, your child's nodes may quickly swell to a peak size in 2 to 3 days and then slowly resolve over 1 to 3 weeks. Once a node has been activated to fight an infection, it will rarely return completely to its original size. Lymph nodes may remain 2 to 3 times as big as their pre-activated size. This is the normal function of a lymph node and is not a cause for concern. Even when there are no health problems, you may still feel small nodes in healthy children. Typically, these benign lymph nodes are easily moved by your fingers from side to side and up and down.

Another very common cause of swollen neck nodes is a strep infection. Infectious mono also causes enlarged neck nodes as well as swollen nodes throughout the body. Some diseases, such as chickenpox, may also cause some of the nodes in the body to swell.

Lymph node enlargement can be present on only one side of the body. For example, if the node swelling is triggered by a cut, usually the nodes only on that side of the body are affected.

Lymph node enlargement in infants less than 2 months of age is unusual, although it may be seen in the head and neck nodes, which drain the scalp of a child with very dry skin, eczema, or scalp abrasions from a traumatic delivery.

There are also more serious causes of lymph node enlargement. For example, lymphoma or childhood leukemia may present with enlarged nodes. Lymph nodes in these instances are generally slow-growing, rarely have an accompanying viral-like illness with fever, may not be easily moved under the skin, may be clumped (matted) together, and are often accompanied by other systemic symptoms such as weight loss and exhaustion.

 ## Expected Course

Most lymph nodes will appear within a day or so of the onset of symptoms such as a sore throat and fever. A small number of nodes may be enlarged at first, but as the illness progresses and your child develops more intense symptoms, more glands are recruited to help fight the infection and the involved glands will become increasingly more swollen. These glands can be quite tender.

In most cases, as the generalized symptoms improve, the glands will shrink back from their peak size to a slightly larger than original size over the next several weeks.

Sometimes there can be surprisingly rapid growth of swollen glands. Parents may report that within a few hours, the neck becomes noticeably swollen. This progression of neck swelling warrants attention. In other instances a single node may increase to a very noticeable size. A single, huge node or a group of nodes that develop redness of the skin overlaying them may also occur. This may mean not only an infection of the lymph node(s), but a spread to the overlaying skin, resulting in a skin infection or cellulitis. Infected nodes are generally much larger, much more tender, and may have redness of the skin overlaying them. This means there is now a bacterial infection as a secondary complication of an initial viral infection. Or, the bacteria (for example, strep) have spread from their original site in the throat to the lymph nodes.

If you are worried about the size and growth of a particular lymph node, you may draw a line around it and check it periodically to see if it has gone beyond the boundaries of the previous margin. This is how we often track the size of an enlarged node.

If a secondary bacterial infection of a lymph node occurs, treatment can usually be managed with outpatient antibiotic therapy. If, however, the growth or redness of the infected node is so rapid, and/or your child appears very ill with high fever and fluid refusal, hospitalization and IV antibiotics may be needed.

If a node or cluster of nodes remains visible and/or grows slowly for several weeks in an otherwise healthy child, please bring that to your health-care provider's attention. Enlarged lymph nodes are almost always caused by an infection—viral or bacterial—but if their presence worries you, it is a good idea to have them checked.

Contagiousness/Immunity

The lymph node itself is not contagious, because it is fully encapsulated and this capsule protects the rest of the body and other children from direct infection exposure. However, the triggering infection that set the process of lymph node enlargement into play may be contagious, certainly if it is viral or strep.

Swollen lymph nodes caused by skin trauma are not contagious.

Home Care

The primary goals of therapy are to provide comfort and to support the body's own immune system as it attempts to attack the invading infectious agent. In addition, it is important to watch carefully for significant increases in node size, any overlaying redness, and more worrisome symptoms. Treatment must also be directed against the triggering event.

We ask you to first read through the entire "Home Care" section to select the recommendations that make the most sense for your child's current situation.

1. Tender lymph node. Ibuprofen or acetaminophen may reduce tenderness. See "OTC Medication Recommendations and Dosages" section. Instruct your child not to repeatedly touch the node, and you should do so infrequently, too. Do not squeeze the node. Placing a warm washcloth or heating pad over the node may provide some relief.

2. Treating the underlying trigger. If a cause is discovered (such as a scrape or bite) or diagnosed (such as an ear infection or strep), get treatment for the underlying cause.

3. Hydration. Good fluid intake is a mainstay for treating all infections and will help to thin and mobilize secretions, providing some relief. This aids the body in clearing infectious agents without stressing the lymph node.

4. Other symptoms. Other symptoms, such as fever, should be treated according to the appropriate sections in the manual.

5. Observation. Take note of the size, color, and relative tenderness of the node site. Repeat your observation every 12 to 24 hours, or sooner if your child's symptoms are worsening.

 ## Integrated Therapies

(Please refer to the section on "Administering Integrated Treatments" on page 19 for guidance on using any of the therapies that follow.)

AROMATHERAPY

- An aromatherapy bath or massage with the essential oils of eucalyptus radiata and/or lavender can soothe and relax your child's anxiety and restlessness. Add 2 to 5 drops of oil to a warm bath and allow your child to soak for a comfortable period of time.

HERBAL REMEDIES (For quick reference please refer to the "Herbal Remedies List" on page 31 and the inside cover.)

- Echinacea/astragalus can be used to support the immune system in helping to resolve a viral infection. For dosing, follow the package labeling accurately.

- Valerian root is a mild herbal sedative that may offer some help in easing a child with significant restlessness. Valerian root may be most useful at bedtime. For dosing, follow the package labeling accurately.

LYMPH NODES (SWOLLEN)

HOMEOPATHIC REMEDIES (For quick reference please refer to the "Homeopathic Remedies List" on page 32 and the inside cover.)

- A homeopathic remedy designed to support the defense system in viral infections may be useful. It can be taken 3 to 6 times daily when the virus is active (for example, fever, lethargy, etc.). (General Support 1)
- A homeopathic remedy designed to decrease inflammation and fever from infections may help prevent deterioration and improve the recovery time. It can be taken 3 to 6 times daily when the virus is active (for example, fever, lethargy, etc.). (General Support 2)
- A homeopathic remedy designed to speed the body's recovery from inflammation may help to minimize swelling and inflammation. It may be taken (1 tablet or 4 drops per dose) 3 to 6 times a day until the inflammation is resolved. (General Support 4)
- A homeopathic remedy designed to relieve acute and severe inflammation may be helpful when given for severe sore throat pain or swollen, tender lymph nodes. It may be taken 3 times daily for up to 3 days. If no relief is achieved within 3 days, you should consult your health-care provider. (General Support 5)

NUTRITIONALS AND SUPPLEMENTS

- Vitamin C
- Zinc

DIETARY GUIDELINES

- It is best to avoid all dairy products and citrus fruits because they may increase or thicken respiratory mucous.
- Reduce or eliminate fried and fatty foods and sugar-sweetened foods from the diet.
- Warm foods such as soups, warm cooked grains (for example, oatmeal), and teas should be given.

INTEGRATIVE SUPPORTIVE CARE

- Please read the section "Integrated Management of Respiratory Illnesses."

 When to Call Your Health-care Provider

Call immediately if any of the following occur:
- The lymph node grows very rapidly.
- Red streaks or redness develops near the node or on the skin overlaying the lymph node.

- Your child becomes progressively more lethargic, difficult to arouse, dehydrated, or inconsolable.
- The lymph node begins to drain pus.

Call within 24 hours if:

- The lymph node slowly reaches 1 to 2 inches in diameter.
- The lymph node becomes very tender to the touch.
- The lymph node remains larger than 1 inch for more than 1 month.
- You suspect a strep infection in a child with a sore throat as well as swollen glands.
- You detect an enlarged node in an infant less than 2 months of age.
- The lymph node seems firmer and more "fixed" in place than on previous observations.
- You detect an enlarged node next to the collar bone.

 ## Other Relevant Sections

Colds

Dehydration

Earache/Ear Infection

First Aid—Bites

First Aid—Cuts and Abrasions

Impetigo

Infectious Mononucleosis

Throat

Integrated Management of Respiratory Illnesses

 ## Prevention

Preventing lymph node enlargement is directly related to preventing the triggering cause. Since most swollen glands are the result of a viral or bacterial infection, careful hand-washing by both child and caregiver is central to prevention. Avoid contact with children known to be ill, especially during high respiratory season. Keep fingernails short to prevent infection from scratching.

Description/Physiology

Nosebleeds are very common in children, especially in dry climates. Tiny blood vessels are very close to the surface of the nasal lining, and may easily break with normal rubbing or picking. These delicate blood vessels are located primarily in the middle wall (septum) of the nose. It may appear as if a good deal of blood has been lost with the average nosebleed, but in reality, only a small amount is usually lost.

 Causes/Epidemiology

Many irritants may predispose to nosebleeds. For example, a cold, allergies with nasal congestion, and even bacterial nasal infections such as impetigo and occasionally sinus infections can create nasal irritation and lead to bleeding.

Many nosebleeds in children are caused by trauma, most commonly from nose-picking but also from a direct external blow to the nose. Once in a while a small child may stick a foreign object up a nostril, which may instantly cause bleeding or, if undetected and stuck in place, may cause a foul-smelling nasal discharge and bleeding from one nostril.

Nosebleeds occur very rarely as the result of a bleeding disorder in which normal blood-clotting is disrupted. A bleeding or clotting disorder may be discovered for the first time, however, because of a difficult-to-control nosebleed. There is often a known family history of a bleeding or clotting disorder.

 Expected Course

Most nosebleeds are benign and short-lived. The usual culprit is the nose-picking child who scratches the membranes of his septum (the inner wall of the nose). Most bleeding is easily controlled with the methods listed below. Some children will awaken with blood on their sheets. While this can be both frightening and unexpected, there is no real danger.

On occasion a nosebleed fails to respond to the recommended methods of treatment. If this is the case, a further evaluation will be required, which could include a visit to your health-care provider, an ENT (Ear, Nose, and Throat) doctor, or a local emergency room to determine the cause of the bleeding and possibly to cauterize the bleeding vessel. This extreme measure is needed in only a tiny fraction of all nosebleeds.

It is rare that the nose is actually broken by trauma. The nose bones are small and very close to the skull, so most of the nose structure itself is cartilage. Nevertheless, nasal trauma, even without a nasal bone fracture, can bleed heavily.

Some children will swallow blood, which, in turn, is irritating to the stomach. This stomach irritation may cause vomiting of the blood, which, while dramatic, is not dangerous. As the swallowed blood is digested, it can also create a black, tarry-appearing stool.

Recurrent nosebleeds are common in some children. If you feel the nosebleeds are too frequent, we recommend that you keep a record of the number of nosebleeds your child has over a several-month period to detect trends, identify obvious triggers, or document an unexpected increase in their frequency. This diary will give you a truly accurate record of the severity and frequency of the nosebleeds as well as enhance your health-care provider's assessment of the problem.

Recurrent nosebleeds may require a direct examination by your health-care provider, blood work, and even a visit to the ENT doctor for additional evaluation. Further investigation is particularly important if there is a family history of a bleeding disorder or if excessive bleeding occurs with other traumatic events such as circumcision, tooth extraction, or routine cuts.

Nosebleeds from high blood pressure are extremely rare in children. Likewise, it is very rare that your child will develop anemia because of frequent nosebleeds.

 ## Contagiousness/Immunity

Nosebleeds are not contagious. However, if a nosebleed is triggered by a viral or bacterial infection in the nasal membranes, these infectious agents are contagious. They will not necessarily produce nosebleeds in another infected child, however.

 ## Home Care

The ultimate goals for treatment of nosebleeds are to control bleeding, provide comfort, calm fears (both child and parent), determine the cause, and work toward prevention. The sight of blood, especially fairly large amounts from the rich blood supply of the nose, can be very frightening to both child and parent. Your calm and comforting manner will reassure your child that everything is under control.

NOSEBLEEDS

We ask you to read through the entire "Home Care" section and select those recommendations that make the most sense for your child's current situation.

1. Have your child sit up and lean forward (rather than lie down or with head tilted). This position reduces swallowing of blood.

2. Firmly, but gently, pinch the entire nose (primarily the soft parts or the lower $^2/_3$ of the nose) against the center wall of the nose (septum) continuously for a minimum of 10 minutes. Press firmly but do not cause further discomfort. Do not be tempted to release the pressure after just a few minutes "to check" whether the bleeding has stopped. Ask your child to breathe through his mouth during this time. At the end of 10 minutes, release gradually and slowly.

   A. Tell your child to relax and breathe through his mouth after pressure has been released. Your gentle reassurance will calm your child's fears and improve cooperation. Sitting near the TV/video or with a book can provide a calming distraction.

   B. If bleeding continues even after 10 minutes of pressure, repeat the pressure for a second 10-minute, continuous period.

   C. If bleeding continues after 3 such attempts, call your health-care provider.

3. A cold washcloth applied to your child's forehead, back of neck, or under the lips generally does not stop a nosebleed. These techniques might instead produce more agitation.

4. Avoid packing your child's bleeding nose with anything (unless your personal experience indicates that this is effective for your child). This is because the packing may initially compress the site of the bleeding, but once the pack is removed it will likely draw the new clot away from the bleeding site and trigger new bleeding.

5. Gently coat the walls of the septum with a thin layer of Neosporin® ointment or Vaseline®. You may do this twice daily. Ocean® Drops or saline drops applied throughout the day may decrease the frequency of nosebleeds.

6. Run a humidifier in your child's bedroom and play area as much of the day and night as possible.

7. Extra hydration with fluids helps keep all mucous membranes moist.

8. Avoid the use of decongestants as they may dry out the moist nasal membranes, making them even more susceptible to irritation and bleeding.

Integrated Therapies

(Please refer to the section on "Administering Integrated Treatments" on page 19 for guidance on using any of the therapies that follow.)

HERBAL REMEDIES (For quick reference please refer to the "Herbal Remedies List" on page 31 and the inside cover.)

- Aloe vera gel can be applied with a cotton swab 2 to 4 times a day to the septum of the nasal cavity (the inner wall of the nostril) to reduce or eliminate nosebleeds.
- Lemon juice can help stop an active nosebleed. Place 1 to 2 drops on a cotton swab and gently rub it onto the septum (the inner wall of the nostril) just inside of the bleeding nostril.

BACH FLOWER REMEDIES

- Rescue Remedy™ may be of use if your child is uncomfortable from the illness, stress, or anxiety. You may use 2 drops every 10 minutes to every few hours to calm restlessness as needed.

NUTRITIONALS AND SUPPLEMENTS

- Vitamin C

 ## When to Call Your Health-care Provider

Call immediately if any of the following occur:

- Bleeding persists after three attempts of holding continuous pressure for 10 minutes.
- The nosebleed is associated with a severe headache.
- The nosebleed is also accompanied by a loss of consciousness from head injury.
- If your child faints because of the nosebleed.
- Anytime a nosebleed follows a tonsillectomy/adenoidectomy.

Call within 24 hours if:

- Bleeding episodes persist off and on over several days or weeks.
- Bleeding is associated with green nasal discharge present for at least 2 weeks.
- You notice any other unusual bruising of your child's skin.

NOSEBLEEDS

 ## Other Relevant Sections

Colds

Hay Fever/Perennial Allergies/Environmental Rhinitis

 ## Prevention

Several of the treatments listed above for an acute nosebleed may be used for prevention, as well. Use a humidifier in your house and in your child's bedroom, running continuously, especially in the winter. Apply Neosporin® ointment, Vaseline®, or aloe vera gel to the nasal septum twice per day. Discourage nose-picking! Trim fingernails closely. Avoid cigarette smoke. Do not use decongestants. Avoid aspirin-containing products.

ROSEOLA

Description/Physiology

Roseola is a relatively common viral illness of childhood. It usually affects children in the 6-month to 4-year age range. Its characteristics are a moderate to high fever (101 to 106 degrees) lasting 2 to 4 days, with very few other symptoms during this time except those brought on by the fever itself, such as irritability, sleep disruption, decreased activity, and poor appetite. Within 24 hours after the fever disappears, the classic roseola rash appears. The roseola rash is a fine, pink rash, mainly on the trunk. The rash may also appear on the face and extremities, but to a much lesser extent. This rash may last several hours to 5 days.

Causes/Epidemiology

Roseola, or roseola infantum, is caused by the human herpes virus type six. The fever and rash of roseola may be confused with measles, but roseola is now far more common than measles because of the measles immunization program.

Roseola occurs throughout the year but has a greater incidence in the spring and summer months. Children of all ages are susceptible, but it is rare to see a case after 4 or 5 years of age. The incubation period after roseola exposure is in the 10- to 15-day range.

Expected Course

As discussed above, roseola first presents with a fever. The fever may range from 101 to 106 degrees, but is usually on the higher end (104 to 106 degrees). The fever can generally be controlled with the measures listed below. There are relatively few other symptoms except those caused by the fever—crankiness, restlessness and agitation, decreased appetite, and disruption of normal sleep pattern. There may be some complaints of achy muscles. Neck glands may be slightly swollen. Children generally self-regulate their activity level. Many sleep more than usual, while others go about their business with little or no notice of the fever.

The fever generally ends abruptly, and within less than 24 hours the lacy, pink, slightly raised, generalized rash appears. This rash can look like a sheet of thousands of small red dots, may feel a bit rough to the touch, and will blanch when pressed. The rash may itch a bit. The rash may remain several more days or resolve within hours after the fever disappears. Usually, the rash of roseola heralds the improvement of your child's illness. Once the fever has broken, most children feel much better and may attempt to return to regular activity.

ROSEOLA

There are very few complications associated with roseola. Naturally, infants with roseola cause more concern because of the high fever and irritability, but even this age group tolerates the virus well.

 ## Contagiousness/Immunity

Roseola is contagious. The virus is spread in the oral and nasal secretions of an infected child. It is not generally transmitted in the air. It may be spread on contaminated fingers. As with most viruses, it can also survive short periods of time on contaminated toys, towels, and books. Careful hand-washing is central to disease prevention.

Roseola is a one-time infection. Thus, like chickenpox, children who acquire roseola once have a lifelong immunity. In addition, there is no risk to the developing fetus should a pregnant woman be exposed to the virus.

Roseola is contagious approximately 24 hours before the fever develops and remains contagious for about 2 to 3 days after the fever has disappeared.

 ## Home Care

Home care is focused on making your child comfortable during the fever phase, isolating your child as much as possible from other children, and essentially riding out the fever and rash. Because it is a viral illness, there is no specific cure.

We ask you to read the entire "Home Care" section and select those recommendations that make the most sense for your child's current situation.

1. Fever: Acetaminophen or ibuprofen may be given for the achiness and irritability caused by the fever. A low-grade fever need not be treated. See "OTC Medication Recommendations and Dosages" section.
   Note: Do not give aspirin to a child with suspected roseola.

2. Hydration: Provide unlimited clear fluids, especially during the fever phase.

3. Activity: Limit your child's activity, especially during the fever. Your child may be surprisingly active even during the fever phase and especially so once the fever has broken and the rash appears. Quiet in-door activity is best. Avoid sun exposure while the rash is present.

4. Sleep: Many children require more sleep than usual. So, provide ample opportunities for sleep in a quiet room with reduced stimulation, and limit out-of-home travel and activities. You may need to be creative with distractions such as books, games, and crafts.

Integrated Therapies

(Please refer to the section on "Administering Integrated Treatments" on page 19 for guidance on using any of the therapies that follow.)

AROMATHERAPY

- An aromatherapy bath or massage with the essential oils of eucalyptus radiata and/or lavender can soothe and relax your child's anxiety and restlessness. Add 2 to 5 drops of oil to a warm bath and allow your child to soak for a comfortable period of time.

HERBAL REMEDIES (For quick reference please refer to the "Herbal Remedies List" on page 31 and the inside cover.)

- Aloe vera or calendula applied topically can reduce itching and soothe irritated skin. They are available in gel, lotion, or cream. For dosing, follow the package labeling accurately.
- Valerian root is a mild herbal sedative that may offer some help in easing a child with significant restlessness. Valerian root may be most useful at bedtime. For dosing, follow the package labeling accurately.

HOMEOPATHIC REMEDIES (For quick reference please refer to the "Homeopathic Remedies List" on page 32 and the inside cover.)

- A homeopathic remedy designed to support the defense systems in viral infections may be useful. It can be taken 3 to 6 times daily when the virus is active (for example, fever, lethargy, etc.). (General Support 1)
- A homeopathic remedy designed to decrease inflammation and fever from infections may help prevent deterioration and improve the recovery time. It can be taken 3 to 6 times daily when the virus is active (for example, fever, lethargy, etc.). (General Support 2)

BACH FLOWER REMEDIES

- Rescue Remedy™ may be of use if your child is uncomfortable from the illness, stress, or anxiety. You may use 2 drops every 10 minutes to every few hours to calm restlessness as needed.
- A lukewarm bath with 10 drops of Rescue Remedy™ added to the bathwater is often very effective at relieving agitation and stress in general.

DIETARY GUIDELINES

- It is best to avoid all dairy products and citrus fruits because they may increase or thicken respiratory mucous.

- Warm foods such as soups, warm cooked grains (for example, oatmeal), and teas should be given.
- Cold foods, foods high in sugar, and fried foods should be avoided.
- Your child may not feel well enough to eat, so don't force food. Instead, make sure that he continues a good intake of fluids and drinks extra water to ensure good hydration. You may use the following table as a general guideline for water in addition to normal fluid intake:

AGE	OUNCES OF WATER PER DAY
2 to 5 years old	12 to 18 ounces
5 to 12 years old	18 to 24 ounces
13 and up	32 to 48 ounces

INTEGRATIVE SUPPORTIVE CARE

- Please read the section "Integrated Management of Respiratory Illnesses."

 When to Call Your Health-care Provider

Call immediately if any of the following occur:
- The rash becomes purple or bluish and spreads rapidly.
- Your child is still lethargic or inconsolable even after ibuprofen or acetaminophen.
- The fever exceeds 105 degrees.
- Your child becomes progressively more toxic looking, with labored breathing, vomiting, and crying with movement.
- Your child has a fever seizure.

Call within 24 hours if:
- Your child's rash lasts more than 5 days.
- The fever recurs once your child begins to feel better.
- Your child develops a sore throat and the rash persists.
- Your child is un-immunized.
- Your child is less than 4 months of age.

Other Relevant Sections

Fever

Hives

Influenza

Throat

Integrated Management of Respiratory Illnesses

 ## Prevention

The best prevention of spread comes with careful hand-washing. Because the virus is most easily spread on contaminated fingers, hand-washing by care providers as well as by the child himself is important. In addition, the infected child should not share utensils, towels, pillowcases, etc. Strict isolation from newborns is advised. Toys and washable items should be washed whenever possible. Healthy children should avoid any child infected with roseola at least until the fever has disappeared and after 2 to 3 days of the appearance of the rash.

Description/Physiology

A bacterial sinus infection is one of the most misunderstood infections in childhood. It is often over-diagnosed both in children and adults. In fact, when exact criteria for the disease are applied, bacterial sinusitis is a surprisingly uncommon diagnosis in children. The long-held public myth has been that any child with a green nasal discharge of any duration, or a headache over the forehead, and/or a cough, automatically has a sinus infection. This is simply not so. In fact, to make the correct diagnosis of a sinus infection in children, certain strict criteria must be met. Most children with mild symptoms of short duration have sinus congestion, not a bacterial sinus infection.

Because there is so much misinformation about sinus infections, we will depart from the usual format of these sections to provide a more comprehensive discussion about its diagnosis. We hope to help you identify when sinus symptoms require medical attention and how to safely treat sinus congestion at home. We recognize that many adults (parents) have a history of sinus infections, but we ask you to view this disease differently in children.

Sinuses are pockets, or cavities, in the skull and facial bones. These cavities are lined by tissues called mucous membranes, which are similar to the membranes that line the inside of the nose. Most of the cavity is filled with air. These cavities drain into the nasal passages by small holes, called ostia.

There are four main sets of sinuses. Each set consists of a right and a left sinus, and they are roughly symmetrical. The two on either side of the nose and behind the cheeks are the maxillary sinuses. The two located behind the eyebrows are the frontal sinuses. Two other sets of sinuses, set deeper in the skull, are the ethmoid and sphenoid sinuses.

The strict definition of "sinusitis" is any inflammatory process of the mucous membranes of the sinuses. The terms sinusitis and bacterial sinus infection are often used interchangeably, but technically that is incorrect. Sinusitis refers to the inflammation of the sinus tissue whether or not it is infected with bacteria. This inflammation is caused by a triggering event. Many triggering events are listed below under "Causes/Epidemiology." These triggers cause an inflammatory response in the mucous membranes of the sinus, resulting in swelling and increased mucous production. The swelling creates a narrowed opening of the ostia, thus slowing the mucous drainage from the sinus. The decreased drainage and increased mucous production lead to sinus congestion.

Sinus congestion commonly occurs as a result of a viral upper respiratory infection (a common cold) or hay fever. The mucous produced by the cold or allergy is unable to flow out of the sinus and thus builds up pressure in the enclosed sinus space, which results in the familiar symptoms. These symptoms may include headache, facial pain, tooth pain, and sinus "pressure."

When bacteria invade the static mucous in the congested sinus, an infection called "bacterial sinusitis" is created. While the symptoms of sinus congestion are commonly mistaken for the diagnosis of a bacterial infection, true bacterial sinusitis is best defined by the color of the nasal discharge and how long the discharge has been present (see below).

Many technological advances, such as the CT scan and MRI studies, have shown that children of all ages may develop sinus infections. However, these studies have also shown that many, if not most, of the children in whom the diagnosis of bacterial sinusitis is made do not actually have a sinus infection at all. The main reason for the frequently incorrect diagnosis of sinus infection: similarities among symptom patterns and characteristics of a sinus infection and symptoms of other problems, the most common of which is sinus congestion from a cold, allergies, or environmental rhinitis.

The key point here is that symptoms such as a thick, green nasal discharge; nasal congestion; persistent hacking cough (especially at night); and low-grade fever are common to many diagnoses, not just bacterial sinusitis. This has led many providers to over-diagnose sinus infection.

This over-diagnosis and treatment of sinus infection has had several negative outcomes. First, patients (and parents) have been trained to believe that a common symptom such as a green nasal discharge is all that is required to establish a diagnosis of true sinus infection. Second, the liberal use of antibiotics has led to a dangerous increase in the presence of antibiotic-resistant strains of bacteria, which makes effective treatment for true sinus infections even more difficult.

Diagnostic Criteria for Sinus Infection

The presence of symptoms listed below is suggestive of bacterial sinusitis, and they warrant further evaluation if they have lingered for more than 14 days. We believe that if the criteria listed below are met, your child has a very high likelihood of having a true sinus infection. If they are not met, there is a high probability that some other diagnosis is the cause of the symptoms, such as environmental rhinitis, viral infection (cold), or allergies.

We feel that for your health-care provider to accurately diagnose a sinus infection, your child must have at least the following minimum criteria:

Group 1: A combination of "criterion a" from Group 1 (see next page) and at least one or more criteria from the rest of Group 1 strongly suggests a sinus infection. While meeting these criteria generally correlates with the diagnosis, the only way to confirm it is by a CT scan.

Group 2: A combination of any three of the four criteria in Group 2 would strongly suggest a true sinus infection.

Group 1

a. Your child has a green nasal discharge, which is usually thick and large in volume, for a minimum of 14 days, without improvement.

b. A deep, congested cough, which is not improving, and, in fact, may be worsening.

c. A dull aching pain over the forehead, face, or upper teeth. This pain may worsen when the child leans forward or bends over.

d. Moderate, if not significant, nasal congestion is present.

e. A low-grade temperature and, on occasion, a high temperature may be present.

Group 2

a. The nasal membranes are abnormal on physical examination and the mucous visible on the upper nasal membranes is green.

b. There is no other diagnosis present that could account for these symptoms.

c. On examination of the throat there is a green postnasal discharge found and a red "cobblestone" appearance of the back of the throat, suggesting chronic drainage with irritation.

d. There is pain on pressing over the facial and forehead sinuses.

 Causes/Epidemiology

Many triggering events are responsible for causing inflammation in the sinuses. In most instances these triggers merely cause inflammation and mild symptoms of sinus congestion that never reach the full-blown sinus infection stage. These triggers include viruses, allergies, air pollution, cigarette and other smoke, strong chemical smells, perfumes, and extremely dry or cold air. There may also be anatomic obstruction of the sinuses, as with large adenoids, that block mucous flow from the sinuses. All of these factors can create an environment conducive to bacterial infections by causing static mucous to accumulate in the sinus.

Expected Course

Your description of your child's symptoms strongly guides your health-care provider to the diagnosis of sinus infection, to decide whether the symptoms are those of a single, lingering cold; two shorter, consecutive colds; or a true sinus infection.

The symptoms of sinus infection may vary according to whether it is acute or chronic as well as with the child's age. With acute sinus infection, children usually have a history of a recent respiratory infection that has worsened or not improved over 2 weeks. Your child may complain of exhaustion and fever. Headache and facial pain may be severe, often worsening when your child bends forward. Pain is most commonly felt in the face and upper teeth. Nasal congestion; thick, green nasal discharge; cough, and bad breath are very common and persistent.

Children with sinus congestion and not sinus infection generally feel better within 5 to 7 days.

Children with sub-acute or chronic sinus infections generally do not have fever. Headache may be present. Fatigue and irritability are common. Earaches and tooth pain may be present. Nasal congestion and runny nose may be minimal; however, posterior nasal drainage, sore throat, throat clearing, and "snorting" are common symptoms. These symptoms may cause restless sleep. There may be bad breath, loss of the sense of smell, and puffiness around the eyes. They usually have a cough, which may increase at night. Chronic sinusitis is diagnosed when a child has these symptoms for longer than 30 days or has had 3 bouts of acute sinusitis over 4 to 6 months.

 Contagiousness/Immunity

The transmission of a bacterial sinus infection to another child is very rare. However, a virus that triggered the process that caused the sinus infection can be contagious. Other triggering events are not contagious, such as allergies, air irritants, etc. Your child may return to school as soon as he is feeling better and the fever has disappeared.

 Home Care

The effective resolution of a sinus infection means more than just sterilizing the bacteria in the infected mucous. The sinus must have a normal balance restored to it, as well. This normal balance means that the sinus is again filled with air instead of mucous and that the inflammation of the membranes lining the sinuses is resolved. Treatment can be classified into the same two categories of acute sinusitis and chronic sinusitis.

The sterilizing of the mucous is the process with which most people are familiar, because it generally requires an antibiotic. However, restoring the sinus to a state of normal balance is not accomplished by the antibiotic; the antibiotic is designed simply to sterilize the mucous of bacteria. It is then the body's job to "heal" the sinus. If the mucous does not drain from the sinus, there is substantial risk of recurrence of sinus infection.

Whether or not the body is able to resolve a sinus infection is directly related to the original triggering cause of the mucous accumulation (for example, allergies) and what is being done to resolve it.

We ask you to read through the entire "Home Care" section to select those recommendations that make the most sense given your child's current situation.

FOR ACUTE SINUSITIS:

1. Sinus pain: Use acetaminophen or ibuprofen. See "OTC Medication Recommendations and Dosages" section.

2. Nasal drainage: Use a nasal saline solution, such as Ocean® Spray. We recommend 2 sprays in each nostril 3 times daily. You may mix your own solution by putting $2^{1}/_{2}$ tsp. of salt in 1 quart of water with 1 tsp. of baking soda. Try to use the saline solution at least 4 times per day with 4 to 5 drops in each nostril. Older children should be encouraged to irrigate their nasal passages.

3. Congestion: Discontinue dairy products for 1 week in children over 1 year of age. Run a vaporizer (cool or warm) in the room while your child sleeps. Elevate the head of the bed when possible.

4. Infection: Antibiotics can help cure the actual bacterial sinus infection. Most of the antibiotics commonly used to treat ear infections are adequate. If this is your child's first bout with sinusitis, a 10-day course is usually sufficient; however, if this is the second or third acute bout, a 3-week course may be recommended. Your health-care provider will advise you of the preferred option.

5. Hydration: Offer your child unlimited amounts of clear liquids to help thin the mucous. Use a vaporizer or humidifier at night.

6. Oral decongestants: We do not recommend them. Based on our clinical experience, we believe they may actually promote thickening of the mucous, making it even less likely to drain.

7. Nasal spray decongestants: These agents may play a role in draining the

sinus and provide symptomatic relief of sinus congestion in the early acute treatment. If a child's congestion or nasal drainage is significant enough to affect his ability to eat, sleep, or rest comfortably, a nasal spray decongestant may be used. Medications such as phenylephrine (Neosynephrine®) or oxymetazoline (Afrin®)* may be used safely. Please see "OTC Medication Recommendations and Dosages" section. These medications also run the risk of causing a "rebound" effect if they are used for a prolonged period of time. A rebound effect means that after the medication has worn off, the symptoms return to a level of severity worse than the original level. Under close medical supervision, they are safe and rebounds are uncommon if the product is used only 2 to 3 times per day for less than 6 days. A general guideline for use is as follows:

AGE	PRODUCT	DOSE AND FREQUENCY (MAXIMUM OF 6 DAYS)
2 to 12 months	$^1/_8$% Phenylephrine	1 to 2 drops, 2 to 3 times/day
1 to 5 years	$^1/_4$% Phenylephrine	1 to 2 drops, 2 to 3 times/day
5 to 12 years	$^1/_2$% Phenylephrine	1 to 2 drops, 2 to 3 times/day
12 and older	1% Phenylephrine	1 to 2 drops, 2 to 3 times/day

*NOTE: When oxymetazoline (Afrin®) is used, change the dose to 1 to 2 times/day for a maximum of 6 days.

For chronic sinusitis:

Despite the use of antibiotics, some children do not have complete resolution of their symptoms. Children may experience some relief with intranasal saline flushes given 3 to 4 times daily. Intranasal steroids may be very helpful. For chronic sinusitis, a minimum of 3 weeks of antibiotics is recommended, and this may extend for as long as 6 weeks, while continuing the above measures.

 ## Integrated Therapies

(Please refer to the section on "Administering Integrated Treatments" on page 19 for guidance on using any of the therapies that follow.)

AROMATHERAPY

- Ravensara aromatica or eucalyptus radiata essential oils may have a preventive effect for sinus infections when used early in the illness. Add 2 to 5 drops of oil to a warm bath and allow your child to soak for a comfortable period of time. You may also add 2 to 3 drops to a tablespoon of a carrier oil and rub into the bottoms of the feet, the chest, and back. It may also be used as a steam inhalation.

SINUS INFECTION

HERBAL REMEDIES (For quick reference please refer to the "Herbal Remedies List" on page 31 and the inside cover.)

- Echinacea/astragalus can be used to support the immune system in helping to resolve a viral infection. For dosing, follow the package labeling accurately.
- Horehound may be very effective in reducing mucous production and thus improve congestion and a wet cough. It may help in the recuperative phase of bronchitis, if there is a significant amount of mucous production. For dosing, follow the package labeling accurately.
- Valerian root is a mild herbal sedative that may offer some help in easing a child with significant restlessness. Valerian root may be most useful at bedtime. For dosing, follow the package labeling accurately.

HOMEOPATHIC REMEDIES (For quick reference please refer to the "Homeopathic Remedies List" on page 32 and the inside cover.)

- A homeopathic remedy designed to support the defense systems in viral infections may be useful. It can be taken 3 to 6 times daily when the virus is active (for example, fever, lethargy, etc.). (General Support 1)
- A homeopathic remedy designed to decrease inflammation and fever from infections may help prevent deterioration and improve the recovery time. It can be taken 3 to 6 times daily when the virus is active (for example, fever, lethargy, etc.). (General Support 2)
- A homeopathic remedy designed to relieve sinus inflammation and drain mucous from the sinuses may be helpful. It can be taken 2 to 6 times a day for 7 to 21 days. (Respiratory 10)
- A homeopathic remedy designed to minimize nasal congestion and mucous, especially when associated with respiratory infections, may be useful. It can be taken 2 to 3 times daily while there is nasal congestion. (Respiratory 3)

BACH FLOWER REMEDIES

- Rescue Remedy™ may be of use if your child is uncomfortable from the illness, stress, or anxiety. You may use 2 drops every 10 minutes to every few hours to calm restlessness as needed.
- A lukewarm bath with 10 drops of Rescue Remedy™ added to the bathwater is often very effective at relieving agitation and stress in general.

NUTRITIONALS AND SUPPLEMENTS

- Vitamin A
- Vitamin C

- Zinc
- Probiotics are especially important to administer during the antibiotic treatment phase and for 2 weeks following the completion of antibiotic therapy.

DIETARY GUIDELINES

- It is best to avoid all dairy products and citrus fruits because they may increase or thicken respiratory mucous.
- Warm foods such as soups, warm cooked grains (for example, oatmeal), and teas should be given.
- Cold foods, foods high in sugar, and fried foods should be avoided.
- Your child may not feel well enough to eat, so don't force food. Instead, make sure that he continues a good intake of fluids and drinks extra water to ensure good hydration. You may use the following table as a general guideline for water in addition to normal fluid intake:

AGE	OUNCES OF WATER PER DAY
2 to 5 years old	12 to 18 ounces
5 to 12 years old	18 to 24 ounces
13 and up	32 to 48 ounces

INTEGRATIVE SUPPORTIVE CARE

- Please read the section "Integrated Management of Respiratory Illnesses."

 When to Call Your Health-care Provider

Call immediately if:

- Sinusitis is rarely a medical emergency and should be dealt with during regular office hours.

Call within 24 hours if:

- From the above description, you suspect that your child has sinusitis, especially with the presence of 14 or more days of green nasal discharge.
- There is redness of the skin overlying the sinuses, and the skin is becoming more red and swollen.
- Sinus pain is so severe that it interferes with sleep.

Other Relevant Sections

Cough

Hay Fever/Perennial Allergies/Environmental Rhinitis

Headache

Nosebleeds

Throat

Integrated Management of Respiratory Illnesses

 ## Prevention

For those children with chronic sinusitis, a combination of environmental changes, diet, and nutritional supplements may be of benefit, as discussed above. You should also teach your child the proper way to blow his nose. Eliminate all known allergens from your child's environment. Avoid contact with cigarette smoke.

STRESS: ITS IMPACT ON YOUR CHILD'S HEALTH

It is no secret that stress has been named as the culprit in many disease processes affecting adults. Numerous studies confirm that children of any age can also be negatively affected by stress. Sleep disorders, eating disorders and obesity, chronic headaches and stomachaches, difficulty with concentration, behavior problems, and depression are just a few of the ailments we see in children who experience chronic stress. In addition, there is strong evidence that the stressed person's body fights off illness less effectively than the body of a person who is in "emotional balance."

Description/Physiology

From primitive times, the human body has been equipped with a "fight or flight" response, originally intended to provide an individual with the extra burst of strength and energy to defend one's self or flee from danger. This physiologic response leads to the excess secretion of hormones and neurotransmitters that lead to secondary changes such as elevated heart rate and blood pressure, anxiety, and/or excitement. In a short "stress" period—for example, the moment just before starting to run a race—the stress response can be beneficial if it sharpens one's senses and promotes optimal performance. Over a prolonged time, however, the effects of a chronic stress response are often detrimental, leading to tension headaches, increased stomach acid secretion and abdominal pain, moodiness and depression. There is also striking evidence that the cells of the immune system function abnormally in individuals who are experiencing chronic stress.

Causes/Epidemiology

Current estimates suggest that as many as 35 percent to 65 percent of children presenting with recurrent abdominal pain or chronic headaches may be suffering from stress in their lives. Reports now point to stress in school rather than heavy backpacks as the primary cause of chronic back pain in middle-school-aged children. Whatever the percentage of children affected by stress, the good news is that identification and treatment is not only possible, but can be quite effective in restoring balance.

265

CAUSES

Parents often correctly intuit that their children experience stress from issues such as marital discord and divorce, parent-child separation, or illness or death of a family member. Often, there can be other causes that are less likely to be suspected:

– infancy and toddler age groups: irregular sleep, poor nutritional habits, hectic life schedules with not enough down time.

– school-aged children: peer problems (such as bullying, exclusion from friends/peer groups, etc.), anxiety associated with learning difficulties and/or test taking, irregular sleep, poor nutritional habits, hectic life schedules with not enough down time.

– adolescents and teens: irregular sleep, poor nutritional habits, hectic life schedules with not enough down time, peer pressures surrounding cliques, appearance, sexual intimidation, substance abuse, and concerns about the safety and well-being of their friends or themselves.

 Expected Course

In the beginning of most cases of stress-related "illness," the symptoms are assumed to be the result of just a common "virus" or "whatever's going around." As the complaints stretch on for days to weeks to months, it becomes clear to the parent that something more must be responsible. That's typically when we are asked to see these children in our office. Often, there is fear that a stomach ulcer or back injury is present. Once a careful history and physical exam can be completed to rule out other causes, reassurance can be given to parent and child, and the possibility of stress can be addressed. Detection of the stressor events can be made; reduction or elimination of the anxiety and the use of "tools" to enhance the child's ability to relax and gain control over his situation can eventually lead to the resolution of his symptoms.

 Home Care

The primary goal of home care is to help you take steps to identify, treat, and prevent the discomfort and imbalance caused by stress-related illness. We ask you to read through the entire "Home Care" section to select those recommendations that make the most sense given your child's current situation.

1. Be sure to refer to the appropriate section in this handbook first (for example, "Headache" or "Abdominal Pain" section).

2. Be tuned in to, accessible to, and involved in your children's day-to-day lives. Get to know what their day is like, who their friends are, what they think of their teachers and coaches, and their performance in the classroom and all activities. All parents are busy, but remember, your children look to you for guidance and acceptance.

3. Keep a diary of symptoms and encourage an older child to do so. Record episodes of "pain," including other details such as date, time of day, location of the pain, activity, what made it better or worse, and associated symptoms. Often, you will both become successful "detectives" as you note a pattern. For example, if the pain is mainly on school days, or after recess, the problem could be a bully intimidating your child.

4. Treat the pain. Just because a symptom is the result of stress, do not assume the pain is "imaginary." The stressed nervous system can produce very "real" discomfort.

   A. For headache/back pain—consider ibuprofen or acetaminophen (see "OTC Medication Recommendations and Dosages" section).

   B. For stomachaches—consider antacids such as Maalox™, Mylanta™, or Tums™ at meals and /or at bedtime, depending upon the timing of the complaint.

5. Sit down with your child to discuss stress in your lives. Depending on his age, you may try different approaches:

   A. Younger children: "What makes you sad?" "What would you wish for?" "Let's draw a picture about your day. Can you tell me about it?"

   B. Older children: Describe how stress makes you feel sometimes. Give examples of stresses you had at that age. Let them know it's not only "OK" to talk about it, but that doing so can lead to a great sense of relief once the stress is "out in the open."

   C. Teens: As above to some extent, but resist the temptation to solve their problems for them. This age group needs not only practice in decision-making and creating strategies for handling conflicts, they also need the confidence gained when parents help support and validate those solutions. Above all, be an empathetic, attentive LISTENER.

6. Regular exercise is a terrific stress reducer. If your child doesn't get daily physical activity, create a plan together and get him moving. Even a period of as little as 20 minutes of exercise can lead to the release of endorphins that promote a feeling of "well-being." Quite often the addition of an after-dinner walk with a parent will open up the

opportunity for conversation about the events of the day.

7. Limit the known stressors you identify in your child's life. Be sure you treat each family member with respect. Marital discord certainly has a great impact on children's stress. Don't place your child in situations he is not yet emotionally ready to handle (for example, coming home to an empty house, staying home alone, dating at an early age). Limit exposure to news, violent and/or inappropriate television, videos, and movies.

8. Become involved in your child's life. Meet and/or speak with your child's teachers on a regular basis. Volunteer in the classroom or simply meet your child at school for a lunch if your school permits, to get a taste of what your child's day is like and how peer interaction plays out there. Be the parent who welcomes your child's friends to your home, the parent who carpools (it's amazing what you hear and learn with a car full of kids!). You'll gain valuable insight into what stresses kids are experiencing today.

9. Minimize your distractions when your child speaks with you. Don't let your cell phone, car radio, TV, etc., ruin an opportunity for your child to speak up.

10. Occasionally, stress can be tougher to handle. That's when the involvement of an experienced child therapist can be of immense help. If your health-care provider suspects counseling may be helpful, they can work with you to refer your child/family to an appropriate therapist.

Integrated Therapies

(Please refer to the section on "Administering Integrated Treatments" on page 19 for guidance on using any of the therapies that follow.)

AROMATHERAPY

- Essential oils, lavender, mandarin, and Roman chamomile will help decrease stress and promote relaxation. These oils may be added to bathwater or dabbed onto "pulse points" beneath the angle of the jaw or the temples of the forehead.

HERBAL REMEDIES (For quick reference please refer to the "Herbal Remedies List" on page 31 and the inside cover.)

- Valerian root may offer some help in easing a child to sleep.

BACH FLOWER REMEDIES

- Rescue Remedy™ may be of use if your child is uncomfortable from stress or anxiety. You may use 2 drops every 10 minutes to every few hours to calm restlessness as needed.
- A lukewarm bath with 10 drops of Rescue Remedy™ added to the bathwater is often very effective for relieving stress in general.
- Bach Flower Remedies™ are a group of homeopathic remedies and can be specifically tailored to your child's individual needs. For further guidance, please consult with your health-care provider.

MASSAGE

- Teach your child with a headache to massage his forehead by using his fingertips, making firm, circular motions. Let him know that he has the power and skill to do this wherever he is, and that he should do so at the FIRST sign of a headache (this will not only help relieve pain by relaxing the muscles of the forehead, but the time spent at that moment will help your child initiate a much-needed period of relaxation).
- Massage your child's feet or back. You may use the oils described above to enhance relaxation.

NUTRITION

- Add a multivitamin to help assure that daily requirements are met.
- Encourage hydration with water on a regular basis.
- Limit intake of caffeine and refined sugars—in many cases it sends kids on a virtual "emotional roller coaster."
- Limit fast food consumption. In general, most of it is high in fat, sodium, sugar, and calories and lower in nutrition.
- Plan and encourage the consumption of regular healthy meals and snacks. Do make an effort to have at least one "family meal" together each day!

 When to Call Your Health-care Provider

Call within 24 hours if:
- Your child's general health, weight gain or loss, or school attendance has been negatively impacted.
- Your child has developed signs of depression.
- You suspect the possibility of an underlying medical problem.

STRESS: ITS IMPACT

🍎 Prevention

Read the suggestions in the "Home Care" section above. Many act as preventive measures!

Pay attention to nutrition and apply regular opportunities for sleep and rest. Avoid "overscheduling" your child. Be sure you teach your child the importance of taking regular time for relaxation every day. That can take the form of yoga, relaxation techniques, meditation, a bath with aromatherapy (see above), listening to or playing music, etc.

Teach your child by your example how to deal with stress. If you make a mistake in how you choose to handle a stressful event, admit that error and describe what you could have done differently. Realize you can be a great example and teacher.

Even if your child no longer needs to be tucked in at night, keep your habit and commitment to touch base with him before you both go to sleep. That private quiet time at the end of the day is often just the opportunity your child needs to share something with you.

Description/Physiology

Sunburn results from overexposure of the skin to the ultraviolet radiation of the sun. A minor sunburn is a first-degree burn that turns the skin pink or red and involves the topmost layer of the skin, the epidermis. Prolonged sun exposure may cause blistering and swelling of the skin and a second-degree burn, in which the epidermis and the underlying layer, the dermis, have been damaged. Sunburn never causes a third-degree burn. Higher altitudes present an even greater risk of sunburn, as ultraviolet (UV) radiation exposure increases at higher elevations.

 ## Causes/Epidemiology

Sunburn is caused by overexposure to ultraviolet radiation. There are two types of UV radiation: Ultraviolet A (UVA) and Ultraviolet B (UVB). Both forms may cause sunburn, although UVA is the more damaging and is especially potent in the summer months. Young children may sustain this skin injury at the beach, at sporting events, while hiking, skiing, and playing outdoors. In adolescents, sunburn may result from time spent in a tanning bed.

In all instances, sunburn is the result of a combination of improper protection of the skin with sunscreen or clothing and excessive exposure to the sun. Sunburn is a serious problem in all children, but especially so in infants who have thin or fair skin. Fair-skinned children need to be protected throughout childhood and even into adulthood. The most common physical characteristics that are predictors for severe sunburn are red or blond hair, blue or green eyes, freckles and/or large numbers of moles.

 ## Expected Course

In most cases, sunburn results in a first-degree burn. Within a few hours after exposure, the skin develops a pink reaction. There may be some skin pain, as well. The pinkness will disappear in a few days with minimal peeling of the skin. Some tanning may occur, as well.

In more extreme cases, which we call second-degree burns, significant redness will develop, and in some instances, blisters. This is especially common on the nose, face, and shoulders. Second-degree burns may be extremely painful, and the pain may last for a number of days. The blisters may rupture, releasing a clear, watery fluid. This degree of burn almost always results in significant peeling of the skin, although it rarely scars. There may be some increased pigmentation in children in the severely sunburned area. Highest risk and often forgotten body areas include the face, especially the ears, lips, nose, and scalp; hands and tops of feet; and shoulders. Your child may not develop more severe reactions until after he has gone to bed.

A very severe sunburn may lead to more serious reactions such as chills, fever, nausea, vomiting, and even mild dehydration. Sunstroke and heat exhaustion are also rare reactions. Heat stroke is characterized by a very high fever (greater than 104 degrees), hot skin, confusion, or loss of consciousness. Heat stroke is the result of dehydration, generally resulting from a combination of inadequate fluid intake and increased fluid loss due to the sun exposure. It can develop very rapidly. Cold and clammy skin, extreme sweating but no fever characterize heat exhaustion. It has a slower onset.

Severe sunburn to the eyes may also occur. The cornea may be damaged, and there may be swelling and edema of the cornea. There can be severe eye pain, temporary blurred or lost vision, and extreme light sensitivity.

 ## Contagiousness/Immunity

This category does not apply for sunburn.

 ## Home Care

The primary goal of home care for sunburn is relief of pain and discomfort. We ask that you please read the entire "Home Care" section and select the recommendations that best fit your child's current situation.

1. Ibuprofen (if your child is older than 6 months) if started early and continued for 2 to 3 days, will reduce pain. See "OTC Medication Recommendations and Dosages" section. Infants less than 6 months may take acetaminophen.

2. Pain symptoms can also be soothed by cool baths, showers, or wet compresses applied several times daily. Baking soda in the bath water may be comforting. Avoid irritating soaps.

3. Peeling may occur within a week. Apply a moisturizing cream during the peeling stage at least twice daily.

4. Offer your child extra water to replace lost fluids.

5. Aloe vera-containing skin-care products are soothing.

6. If your child develops itching as the sunburn heals or peels, a short course of an antihistamine such as Benadryl® may help.

7. Anesthetic skin sprays that contain benzocaine, such as Solarcaine®, may be of some value.

8. Open blisters should be treated with a thin layer of an antibiotic ointment (OTC), such as Neosporin® or Bacitracin.

 ## Integrated Therapies

(Please refer to the section on "Administering Integrated Treatments" on page 19 for guidance on using any of the therapies that follow.)

AROMATHERAPY

- Lavender essential oil sprayed on as a skin wash can be very effective in relieving the discomfort as well as promoting healing of sunburned skin. To make a lavender skin wash, add 10 drops of therapeutic grade lavender oil to 1 to 2 ounces of purified water and apply 3 to 4 times a day from a spray bottle.

HERBAL REMEDIES (For quick reference please refer to the "Herbal Remedies List" on page 31 and the inside cover.)

- Aloe vera applied topically can reduce itching and soothe irritated skin as well as promote healing. A gel of pure aloe is probably the best topical product to use. Lotion or cream with aloe is an acceptable second choice.

- Calendula is also an excellent way to promote healing after the initial burn has responded to aloe. Creams or lotions may be applied 2 to 3 times per day for 1 to 2 weeks after the burn.

- Valerian root is a mild herbal sedative that may offer some help in easing a child with significant restlessness or pain. Valerian root may be most useful at bedtime. For dosing, follow the package labeling accurately.

HOMEOPATHIC REMEDIES (For quick reference please refer to the "Homeopathic Remedies List" on page 32 and the inside cover.)

- A homeopathic cream designed to soothe inflamed or irritated skin may be useful. It can be applied directly to the affected area 3 times a day. (Skin 1)

- A homeopathic remedy designed to reduce the symptoms of skin irritation and breakdown may promote healthy skin. It can be taken 2 to 3 times daily for up to 2 weeks until the skin is completely healed. (Skin 2)

- A homeopathic remedy designed to decrease inflammation may help prevent deterioration and improve the recovery time. It can be taken 3 to 6 times daily in the early days of the burn healing. (General Support 2)
- A homeopathic remedy designed to speed the body's recovery from inflammation may help minimize swelling and inflammation. It may be taken (1 tablet or 4 drops per dose) 3 to 6 times a day until the inflammation is resolved. (General Support 4)

BACH FLOWER REMEDIES

- Rescue Remedy™ may be of use if your child is uncomfortable from the illness, stress, or anxiety. You may use 2 drops every 10 minutes to every few hours to calm restlessness as needed.
- A lukewarm bath with 10 drops of Rescue Remedy™ added to the bathwater is often very effective at relieving agitation and stress in general.

NUTRITIONALS AND SUPPLEMENTS

- Vitamin A
- Vitamin C
- Vitamin E can be used topically to speed skin healing and minimize scarring. Poke a hole in a Vitamin E gel cap and then squeeze some into the palm of your hand and gently rub it directly onto burned area. This may be done once or twice daily.

DIETARY GUIDELINES

- Good fluid intake is essential to healing any sunburn as well as preventing dehydration in more severe cases. You may use the following table as a general guideline for water in addition to normal fluid intake:

AGE	OUNCES OF WATER PER DAY
2 to 5 years old	12 to 18 ounces
5 to 12 years old	18 to 24 ounces
13 and up	32 to 48 ounces

When to Call Your Health-care Provider

The tips suggested here will nearly always be sufficient to manage even severe sunburn.

Call immediately if any of the following occur:
- Pain is so severe that your child is inconsolable.
- Your infant is significantly sunburned, especially on the face.
- Your child is dehydrated and very lethargic. See "Dehydration" section.
- Your child's face is very swollen and badly blistered.
- Your child passes out or is too weak to sit or stand.
- Your child develops severe eye pain, extreme light sensitivity and/or blurred vision or partial blindness.

Call within 24 hours if:
- The sunburn becomes infected and begins to ooze a pus-like drainage.
- Your child is still very irritable, especially an infant.

 Other Relevant Sections

First Aid—Burns

 Prevention

Sunburn is an avoidable childhood problem, but its prevention requires constant vigilance on the part of parents. Assume that every day is a sun exposure day and be prepared at all times for preventive measures. Keep a bottle of sunscreen in the diaper bag, soccer/sport bag, ski parka, car, etc., so you will always be ready.

The most important reason to prevent sunburn, besides the obvious discomfort, is to prevent skin cancer later in life. Although skin cancer occurs almost exclusively in adults, it is triggered by repeated sun exposure and sunburns in childhood. The most extreme sunburns are the highest risk triggers for skin cancer. Every time you apply sunscreen to your child's skin, you are helping prevent skin cancer later in life. Secondarily, sunburn prevention also reduces accelerated damage and aging of the skin.

SUNBURN

HERE ARE SOME HELPFUL PREVENTIVE TIPS:

1. Apply sunscreen every time your child is going outside for more than 30 minutes. An SPF (Sun Protection Factor) of 15 or greater is recommended.
2. Try to keep sun exposure to small increments early in the season until an underlying protective tan builds up.
3. Children with the least skin pigment must be instructed to repeatedly use a sunscreen throughout the year and to avoid the sun whenever possible.
4. The skin of infants is thin and very sensitive to the sun's rays. Sunscreens, protective clothing, and a hat with a brim are essential for an infant's protection. Do not use a sunscreen containing PABA for infants less than 6 months of age. Watch out particularly for the face, hands, and tops of feet. Infants should remain in shade at all times except during the earliest and latest hours of daylight. Even then, sun exposure should be minimal.
5. Especially avoid sun exposure during the hours of 10 a.m. to 3 p.m., when the sun's rays are most intense and damaging.
6. Don't let overcast days fool you. Most of the sun's UV rays still penetrate clouds.
7. Reflection of the sun's rays off water, sand, and snow also increase the risk of sunburn. The shade from a hat or umbrella may not always protect your child from reflected rays. Suntan oils and lotions without sunscreen also magnify the sun's ultraviolet rays.
8. Protect your child's eyes. Years of eye exposure to ultraviolet light increase the risk of cataracts. Buy sunglasses with ultraviolet (UV) protection. Sunglasses will also help prevent acute damage to the cornea.
9. Set a good example. Did you apply your sunscreen, too? Do your sunglasses have UV protection?
10. Remind your adolescents over and over again about the dangers of sunburn. Discourage their preoccupation or obsession with tanning. Discourage tanning bed use.

SUNSCREENS

There are many good sunscreens on the market that prevent sunburn but still permit gradual tanning to occur. The sun protection factor (SPF) or filtering power of the product determines what percent of the ultraviolet rays get through to the skin. The SPF of various products ranges from 2 to 45.

For practical purposes, in an average child, an SPF higher than 30 is rarely needed, because sun exposure beyond five hours is unusual. Although children with more skin pigment probably do not need the higher levels of SPF, as a general rule, we recommend that children receive a sunscreen of at least SPF 15. Children at higher risk for burning, very fair skinned and fair-haired children, should receive a sunscreen of SPF 30.

The most common reason for sunburn while using adequate SPF protection is failure to use enough sunscreen. You should apply liberally, using about 1 ounce of sunscreen for an adult-sized person and proportionately less for your child.

Apply sunscreen 30 minutes before exposure to the sun to allow time for its penetration into the skin. Give special attention to the areas most likely to be exposed. Most products need to be reapplied every 2 to 3 hours, as well as immediately after swimming or profuse sweating. A "waterproof" sunscreen stays on a child's skin only about 30 minutes in water. Be sure to take advantage of opportunities to re-apply sunscreen hourly at the pool or beach.

To prevent sunburned lips, apply a lip coating that also contains PABA. If your child's nose or some other area has been repeatedly burned during the summer, protect it completely from all the sun's rays with zinc oxide ointment.

PABA-containing sunscreens are not recommended for children under 6 months. A good PABA-free sunscreen suitable for babies is Water BABIES®.

SWIMMER'S EAR

 ## Description/Physiology

Swimmer's ear, also called otitis externa, is an infection of the skin of the ear canal. It is a relatively common childhood problem, characterized by itchy, occasionally painful, and draining ear canals. It is distinctly different from an "otitis media" ear infection, which is an infection of the middle ear space, beyond the eardrum (please see the "Ear Infection" section). Children most prone to swimmer's ear are those who spend lots of time in the water, such as swimmers or children who spend a great deal of time in the bathtub or hot tubs.

 ## Causes/Epidemiology

Swimmer's ear is an infection of the skin that lines the ear canal. The ear canal begins just inside the ear itself. This canal leads down to the eardrum. When water gets trapped in the normally dry ear canal, especially if the water contains chlorine or other irritating chemicals, the ear canal lining becomes inflamed, swollen, and prone to infection.

Bacteria—which live normally on the intact, dry skin of the ear canal— penetrate into deeper skin layers because of the inflamed disruption of the normal skin barrier. The inflammation triggers a clear mucous production, followed by a thicker, yellow, pus-like drainage that oozes or pours out of the ear canal.

 ## Expected Course

The typical picture is a child who swims often and who begins to complain that his ears are "itchy." You may witness your child putting his fingers in the ear canals and rubbing them vigorously even before complaining of pain or itching. There may be a red irritation at the ear opening, as well.

This itching is usually followed by the production of a clear discharge and then a yellow drainage. There can be a considerable volume of drainage. At this stage there will usually be some degree of pain involved, as well. Frequently, there will be pain when the outer ear is gently moved up and down. Children will often complain that they cannot hear well or that sounds are muffled, because their ear canals are plugged with mucous.

Once a diagnosis is made, swimmer's ear is treated quite easily, and your child can expect relief within 1 or 2 days.

Yellow pus drainage in the presence of fever, pain, and irritability may also be the result of a ruptured eardrum. This distinction may be difficult without your health-care provider's direct examination, and the treatments for otitis media and swimmer's ear are very different.

 ## Contagiousness/Immunity

Swimmer's ear is not contagious. Some children are especially prone to recurrent swimmer's ear. There is no immunity conferred by previous infection.

 ## Home Care

The goal of home care is to relieve the itching, plugged-ear sensation, and pain that plague your child.

We ask you to first read through the entire "Home Care" section to select which recommendations make the most sense in your child's current situation.

1. You may use acetaminophen or ibuprofen for relief of mild discomfort. See "OTC Medication Recommendations and Dosages" section.

2. Your child should not swim until the symptoms are gone.

3. Do not use earplugs for prevention or treatment unless recommended by your health-care provider or an ear specialist. Earplugs may force earwax deeper into the ear canal. For the same reason, cotton swabs should not be inserted into ear canals.

 ## Integrated Therapies

(Please refer to the section on "Administering Integrated Treatments" on page 19 for guidance on using any of the therapies that follow.)

HERBAL REMEDIES (For quick reference please refer to the "Herbal Remedies List" on page 31 and the inside cover.)

- Valerian root is a mild herbal sedative that may offer some help in easing a child with significant restlessness or pain. Valerian root may be most useful at bedtime. For dosing, follow the package labeling accurately.

- Willow bark extract may help an earache as a topical pain reliever. Place 2 to 3 drops in the painful ear (or both ears) and place a cotton plug in the ear canal to keep the drops from draining out. This should be repeated as often as every 2 to 4 hours. Warm the oil each time.

SWIMMER'S EAR

HOMEOPATHIC REMEDIES (For quick reference please refer to the "Homeopathic Remedies List" on page 32 and the inside cover.)

- A homeopathic remedy designed to speed the body's recovery from inflammation may help minimize swelling and inflammation. It may be taken (1 tablet or 4 drops per dose) 3 to 6 times a day until the inflammation is resolved. (General Support 4)

BACH FLOWER REMEDIES

- Rescue Remedy™ may be of use if your child is uncomfortable from the illness, stress, or anxiety. You may use 2 drops every 10 minutes to every few hours to calm restlessness as needed.

 When to Call Your Health-care Provider

Swimmer's ear is not an emergency. Other ear problems are described in the "Ear Infection" section.

Call within 24 hours if:

- The symptoms have not improved within 5 days of treatment.
- The ear pain worsens 24 hours after beginning treatment.
- The lymph nodes in front of the ear or behind the ear lobe become swollen and tender.
- The ear itself becomes swollen, red, tender to the touch, or is pushed forward.

 Other Relevant Sections

Earache/Ear Infection

 Prevention

The key to prevention is keeping ear canals dry. After your child swims, drain water out of his ear canals by turning his head to the side and gently pulling the ear lobe in different directions to help the water run out. Carefully dry the opening to the ear canal.

For the child prone to swimmer's ear you may also try a drop of the antibiotic eardrops after swimming as a preventive measure. In addition, 2 to 3 drops of rubbing alcohol or specific drops (which can be purchased OTC at the pharmacy or sports store) can be instilled in the ear canals each time after he swims. You may also use a blow-dryer on cool/low setting to dry the ears, with great caution to avoid burning your child. Special earplugs can also be made that prevent water from getting into the ear canal during swimming.

TEETHING

 Description/Physiology

"Teething" refers to the process of the baby's first teeth migrating up from the deep part of the gums to the surface. It can be associated with drooling and chewing. This process is difficult to diagnose because there are no visible changes in the gums, so it is difficult to know if teeth are moving. "Cutting teeth" refers to the process of the tooth actually erupting through the gum surface. If the cutting teeth are surrounded by mild inflammation, there can be associated irritability, low fever (no greater than 101 degrees rectal), mild diarrhea, runny nose, sleep disruption, and some loss of appetite. It's impossible to predict when the "teething" process will result in the "cutting" of a tooth.

 Causes/Epidemiology

The timing of teething is genetically determined and is "switched on" at the appropriate time by the body's own biological clock. There is no way to alter the process. It has been noted that siblings have similar timing patterns for teething, but this is certainly not universally so.

 Expected Course

Your baby's first tooth may appear anytime between the ages of 3 months and 1 year. It is very uncommon for a child not to have at least one tooth before 18 months. The first teeth to erupt are usually the lower middle teeth. You can expect roughly one tooth on average per month until all 20 baby teeth are in place. This is usually completed by $2^1/_2$ years.

You will notice that your generally happy baby begins to have periods during the day when he is crabby, puts everything in his mouth, drools excessively and may also have a low fever (no greater than 101 degrees), mild diarrhea, runny nose, sleep disruption, and some loss of appetite. The process of teething may last a number of weeks until a tooth finally erupts. Because it is normal behavior for infants to drool and put things in their mouth, drooling and mouthing aren't always associated with cutting teeth.

Because so many teeth erupt during the first two years of life, it may appear as if your child is in a constant state of teething. To some extent this is true. Some children are quite affected by the tooth eruption process, while others cut a tooth and there are no indications until the tooth appears. It is rare that teething produces significant symptoms that require medical attention. On occasion, just as the tooth is about to erupt through the gum, a blood blister will form under the surface of the gum. This blister will disappear once the tooth has fully erupted.

It is often noted that molars are a bit more painful to erupt than the other teeth. This may or may not be true in an individual child, but they certainly do take longer to complete the eruption process.

Teething can lead to an increased production of mucous and congestion, which may predispose a child to an ear infection.

Your child's permanent teeth begin to erupt in the age range of 5 to 7 years. These permanent teeth act to push out the baby teeth. There is less pain associated with the eruption of permanent teeth.

 ## Contagiousness/Immunity

This section does not apply to teething.

 ## Home Care

Our primary goals for management of cutting teeth are to control discomfort, provide good hydration, and preserve sleep. Any combination of the following may be required to achieve these goals.

We ask you to first read through the entire "Home Care" section and select those recommendations that make the most sense for your child's situation.

1. For the discomfort associated with teething, use acetaminophen or ibuprofen. See "OTC Medication Recommendations and Dosages" section. Ibuprofen is fine after 6 months of age.

2. For general discomfort and irritability, cut bananas, pears, or similar fruits into large sticks and freeze them. Allow your baby to chew on the frozen fruit. This freezing action on the gums may help numb them, while the chewing may assist the tooth to erupt. Rubbing the gums with an ice cube may help, or try a frozen bagel for chewing. Avoid any hard foods that your baby might choke on.

3. Over-the-counter teething medications (for example, Orajel®) are generally ineffective because drooling washes them out of your baby's mouth very quickly. Also, they expose your infant to the topical anesthetic, benzocaine, numbing ingredient. Benzocaine may actually numb the throat in addition to the gums and may make it difficult for your child to handle his own saliva. In general, we do not recommend over-the-counter teething medications.

4. Distraction or diverting your child's attention often lets him "forget about the pain." Books, toys, car rides, and videos are all good distraction techniques.

5. A teething ring or pacifier, especially if chilled in the refrigerator or in ice water, may help. To avoid the risk of choking, do not tie the teething ring around your child's neck. For chewing, a wet washcloth that has been in the freezer affords some relief.

6. T.L.C. is sometimes the only thing that really helps!

7. At night, Benadryl® may help. See "OTC Medication Recommendations and Dosages" section. This is an antihistamine preparation and may make your child sleepy. We recommend this only after other home-care options have been tried.

8. Gentle massage of the gums for 2 minutes may help.

 ## Integrated Therapies

(Please refer to the section on "Administering Integrated Treatments" on page 19 for guidance on using any of the therapies that follow.)

AROMATHERAPY

- An aromatherapy bath or massage with the essential oils of eucalyptus radiata and/or lavender can soothe and relax your child's restlessness. Add 2 to 5 drops of oil to a warm bath and allow your child to soak for a comfortable period of time.

HERBAL REMEDIES (For quick reference please refer to the "Herbal Remedies List" on page 31 and the inside cover.)

- Valerian root is a mild herbal sedative that may offer some help in easing a child with significant restlessness or pain. Valerian root may be most useful at bedtime. For dosing, follow the package labeling accurately.

HOMEOPATHIC REMEDIES (For quick reference please refer to the "Homeopathic Remedies List" on page 32 and the inside cover.)

- A homeopathic remedy designed to relieve symptoms associated with teething may be helpful. It may be given 3 to 6 times per day during times of tooth eruption. (Pain 4)

- A homeopathic remedy designed to speed the body's recovery from inflammation may help to minimize swelling and inflammation. It may be taken (1 tablet or 4 drops per dose) 3 to 6 times a day until the inflammation is resolved. (General Support 4)

BACH FLOWER REMEDIES

- Rescue Remedy™ may be of use if your child is uncomfortable from the illness, stress, or anxiety. You may use 2 drops every 10 minutes to every few hours to calm restlessness as needed.
- A lukewarm bath with 10 drops of Rescue Remedy™ added to the bathwater is often very effective at relieving agitation and stress in general.

 When to Call Your Health-care Provider

Teething is not an emergency. Therefore, all calls can be held until the following morning.

Parents and providers alike may presume that mild symptoms as described above are only teething. If these symptoms worsen or new symptoms develop, however, it is prudent to follow further instructions in this book, based on new symptoms that develop, and call your health-care provider when appropriate.

Call within 24 hours if:
- Your child's discomfort becomes increasingly more difficult to control.
- The fever exceeds 102 degrees or your child becomes lethargic.

 Prevention

Teething is a natural biological milestone and as such cannot be prevented. Teething symptoms can, however, be helped.

Prevention practices for dental decay in children are directed toward good oral hygiene. Before 1 year of age, warm, wet gauze may be used to gently rub the gums free of any food particles and early plaque. After 1 year, you should brush your child's teeth at least twice daily with a very soft toothbrush. In general, toothpaste is not recommended unless it is specifically designated as baby-safe.

Your child should be instructed at an early age to begin to brush his own teeth. There are toothbrushes designed for small children. In general, any commercial toothpaste without fluoride is fine for your child. There are, of course, children's toothpastes, so the choice is yours. Most dentists recommend the first dental evaluation between 2 and 3 years. Toothpaste with fluoride is recommended for children ten years of age or older.

SORE THROAT/PHARYNGITIS
STREP THROAT
TONSILLITIS

 ## Description/Physiology

A sore throat is a very common symptom in childhood. Most sore throats are triggered by a viral infection as part of a cold syndrome, and only a small percentage are caused by a bacterial infection such as strep. There are many other causes as discussed below.

A sore throat is rarely an isolated symptom. Depending on the cause, there may be a cough, fever, congestion, runny nose, or disruptions of sleep and appetite.

Sore throats are caused by an inflammatory reaction in the tissues of the throat. As it is often the first line of defense, the throat becomes inflamed from being exposed to inhaled irritants (cigarette smoke), allergens, infectious agents, etc.

A sore throat can be divided into four anatomical categories:

1. Pharyngitis: Inflammation of the throat behind the tongue.

2. Tonsillitis: Inflammation of the tonsils.

3. Laryngitis: Inflammation of the larynx (voice box).

4. Tracheitis: Inflammation of the trachea.

Inflammation may be present in all four areas simultaneously. The throat is also the pathway of drainage for a number of head structures, including the nose, sinuses, and upper airway.

The body may handle an invading infectious agent with very few symptoms—in other words, the body's own immune system can clear the agent in just a few short days. However, depending on how aggressive the infection or irritants are, inflammation may evolve rapidly, resulting in swelling of the soft tissue structures, mucous production, and pain. Many infections trigger swollen lymph nodes, which are the body's immune system sites where mucous and debris from the inflamed throat are processed (see "Lymph Nodes or Swollen Glands").

Some infections have a predilection for certain parts of the throat. For example, the croup virus affects the soft tissues around the voice box and trachea. Strep often attacks the tonsils and the tissues in the upper throat. Inhaled irritants will affect whichever tissues they contact.

Causes/Epidemiology

There are a multitude of causes for sore throat. One of the most common are viruses that trigger a common cold. There are dozens of viruses in a single season that are capable of producing a cold and sore throat. Other viruses such as infectious mononucleosis are known for producing a sore throat, as well. In addition, certain bacteria target the throat. Typically, strep infections cause sore throat, fever, abdominal pain, and rash.

Other causes of sore throat include allergies, a dry climate, injury to the throat, chronic sinus congestion or infection, postnasal drip, and irritation from a cough (acute or chronic). Children who sleep with their mouths open may awaken in the morning with a dry mouth and sore throat. Children with a postnasal drip from any cause, including draining sinuses, allergies, etc., may have a sore throat from frequent throat-clearing.

 ## Expected Course

How long the sore throat lasts depends on the causative agent, the age of the child, the intensity of the illness, accompanying symptoms, and the general immune health of the child.

Very young children cannot complain specifically about a sore throat, but may demonstrate decreased appetite, put fingers in their mouth, drool, pull at the muscles in their neck, act irritable, and cry during feedings.

Symptoms of a typical viral sore throat usually last 3 to 5 days. The onset of pain may be gradual or abrupt, with a peak of pain around the third day and gradual improvement thereafter. There is often an accompanying fever, swelling of the lymph nodes in the neck, irritability, loss of appetite, restless sleep, and agitation. Viral sore throats are often mild, but severe pain may also result. The sore throat of mono may be especially debilitating and protracted. The swelling may affect breathing and may intensify snoring. Depending on the original size of the tonsils, there may be enough swelling to appear to make breathing uncomfortable. There may be pus on the tonsils, as well.

"Strep" throat is often associated with headache, fever, a red sandpaper-like rash or hives, swollen neck glands, large tonsils with "pus pockets," and occasionally abdominal pain. Strep throat is uncommon in children under 2 years of age. Oftentimes you will be alerted to a strep exposure at school or daycare. Some children with strep infections may develop "scarlet fever." This variation of strep is characterized by all of the symptoms of strep throat and a classic red, slightly raised, and sandpaper-feeling rash, spread out across the body. This rash can last up to one week and the skin may peel after that.

Other head and neck infections may cause a sore throat as a secondary symptom. For example, in a sinus infection, ear infection, or nasal infection, mucous drainage passing through the throat can be irritating to the throat structures.

Some throat infections may lead to more serious complications. For example, an abscess in the tonsillar area may develop. Stridor may develop in the child with advanced croup. See "Croup" section. Epiglottitis, an inflammation of the epiglottis (a structure that protects the airway), is a serious bacterial infection with an abrupt onset that may act very much like croup.

Other triggers, such as dry climates, are very common. Allergies may cause throat inflammation and mucous production and contribute to a postnasal drip which itself irritates the throat.

Recurrent sore throats are common, especially in children with large tonsils. Recurrent tonsillitis, strep infections, and croup may warrant additional evaluation by your health-care provider as well as by an ENT (Ear, Nose, and Throat) doctor. Tonsillectomy, although a relatively uncommon procedure in children nowadays, may be recommended if specific criteria are met.

Contagiousness/Immunity

Sore throats are contagious only if an infectious agent, a virus, or bacteria cause them. The mechanism of transmission is both through the air and through oral and nasal secretions passed from one infected child or adult to another, usually through direct hand contact.

A child may develop an immunity to one type of virus and not be re-infected with that virus; however, one viral infection does not confer immunity against all the other viruses active in the community during a particular season. With a viral infection, your child is generally no longer contagious and may return to school when the fever has disappeared for 24 hours and other symptoms have been relieved, so that your child has the energy to return to school.

A single strep infection does not create immunity, either. It is rare to see strep before the age of 2 years, although it can be seen even in this age group if there is a very close exposure, such as with a sibling or parent.

Some children may never contract strep, despite close exposure. Others may contract strep readily with exposure. In addition, there may be a "carrier state" in which the child carries the strep infection in his throat but does not have active symptoms. This child is contagious to others but is not actually infected. This diagnosis requires an office visit and specific lab tests. The only way to accurately diagnose strep is with a throat culture or with a "Rapid Strep Test." If the infection is strep, treatment should include symptomatic relief as described below, as well as an antibiotic.

The primary reasons for treating strep with antibiotics are: (1) antibiotics prevent contagion after 24 hours of use, and (2) antibiotics have been shown to prevent two primary late complications of strep throat (a heart disease called rheumatic fever and an inflammatory disease of the kidney).

Contrary to popular belief, antibiotics do not always improve early symptoms or hasten recovery from strep. Much of your child's symptom relief comes from his own immune system fighting off the infection.

After taking antibiotics for 24 hours, your child with strep is no longer considered contagious. He may return to school when the fever is gone and he is generally feeling better.

Home Care

The goals of home care are to provide comfort, relieve pain, ensure good hydration, and support the body's own immune system until the underlying cause has been resolved.

Many of the treatments for symptoms that accompany a sore throat may also relieve the sore throat itself. See "Colds," "Fever," "Cough," and "Lymph Node" sections.

We ask you to first read the entire "Home Care" section and select the recommendations that make the most sense given your child's current situation.

1. Acetaminophen or ibuprofen. See "OTC Medication Recommendations and Dosages" section. Ibuprofen is not for use in children less than 6 months of age. In general, ibuprofen probably works better to relieve sore throat pain than acetaminophen. Do not give aspirin or aspirin-containing products to your child.

2. Sore throat pain can be most difficult to relieve, but along with the pain relievers listed above, throat lozenges (for example, Original Ricola® Herbal Cough Drops) or "hard" candy (such as butterscotch) all provide throat-soothing protection. There is also a variety of herbal teas that soothe throat pain when sipped (for example, Throat Coat® Tea by Traditional Medicinals). OTC throat sprays such as Chloraseptic® or Super Kids Throat Spray™ by Herbs for Kids may also provide some relief. (For dosing, follow package directions accurately.)

3. Distraction often provides remarkable relief. Books, video games, stories, and puzzles may help take your child's mind off the pain.

4. Warm, saltwater gargles for children over 8 years of age may be helpful. Gargling with an antacid may provide coating relief.

5. Good hydration, especially with cool, clear liquids, helps. Dairy products should be avoided because of their mucous-producing tendencies. Keep a water bottle nearby at all times. Popsicles and warm soups may also be soothing.

6. Run a humidifier or vaporizer in the bedroom or play area. Cool mist is preferable.

7. Keep the head of the bed elevated as this allows better mucous drainage at night.

8. Do not use leftover antibiotics.

9. Lots of rest with limited activity will help focus the body's resources on healing and not playing.

10. Keep your child away from cigarette smoke.

11. Provide a soft diet that is bland: avoid spicy, citrus, and salty foods that may be painful to swallow.

 ## Integrated Therapies

(Please refer to the section on "Administering Integrated Treatments" on page 19 for guidance on using any of the therapies that follow.)

AROMATHERAPY

- An aromatherapy bath or massage with the essential oils of eucalyptus radiata and/or lavender can soothe and relax your child's anxiety and restlessness. Add 2 to 5 drops of oil to a warm bath and allow your child to soak for a comfortable period of time.

HERBAL REMEDIES (For quick reference please refer to the "Herbal Remedies List" on page 31 and the inside cover.)

- Valerian root is a mild herbal sedative that may offer some help in easing a child with significant restlessness or pain. Valerian root may be most useful at bedtime. For dosing, follow the package labeling accurately.

- Horehound may be very effective in reducing mucous production and thus may help sore throat pain caused by postnasal drip. It may help in the recuperative phase of throat infections, especially if there is a significant amount of mucous production. For dosing, follow the package labeling accurately.

HOMEOPATHIC REMEDIES (For quick reference please refer to the "Homeopathic Remedies List" on page 32 and the inside cover.)

- A homeopathic remedy designed to support the defense system in viral infections may be useful (not to be used when the diagnosis is strep throat). It can be taken 3 to 6 times daily when the virus is active (for example, fever, lethargy, etc.). (General Support 1)
- A homeopathic remedy designed to decrease inflammation and fever from infections may help prevent deterioration and improve the recovery time. It can be taken 3 to 6 times daily when the virus is active (for example, fever, lethargy, etc.). (General Support 2)
- A homeopathic remedy designed to relieve some of the discomfort associated with infections (for example, fever, body aches, chills, and fatigue) may be useful. It can be taken 3 to 6 times daily when the virus is active (for example, fever, lethargy, etc.). (General Support 3)
- A homeopathic remedy designed to relieve acute and severe inflammation may be helpful when given for severe sore throat pain or swollen, tender lymph nodes. It may be taken 3 times daily for up to 3 days. If no relief is achieved within 3 days, you should consult your health-care provider. (General Support 5)

BACH FLOWER REMEDIES

- Rescue Remedy™ may be of use if your child is uncomfortable from the illness, stress, or anxiety. You may use 2 drops every 10 minutes to every few hours to calm restlessness as needed.
- A lukewarm bath with 10 drops of Rescue Remedy™ added to the bathwater is often very effective at relieving agitation and stress in general.

NUTRITIONALS AND SUPPLEMENTS

- Vitamin A
- Vitamin C
- Zinc

DIETARY GUIDELINES

- Reduce or eliminate fried and fatty foods and sugar-sweetened foods from the diet.
- Warm foods such as soups, warm cooked grains (for example, oatmeal), and teas should be given.
- It is best to avoid all dairy products and citrus fruits because they may increase or thicken respiratory mucous.

- Eliminate caffeine intake.
- Your child may not feel well enough to eat, so don't force food. Instead, make sure that he continues a good intake of fluids and drinks extra water to ensure good hydration. You may use the following table as a general guideline for water in addition to normal fluid intake:

AGE	OUNCES OF WATER PER DAY
2 to 5 years old	12 to 18 ounces
5 to 12 years old	18 to 24 ounces
13 and up	32 to 48 ounces

INTEGRATIVE SUPPORTIVE CARE

- Please read the section "Integrated Management of Respiratory Illnesses."

 When to Call Your Health-care Provider

Call immediately if any of the following occur:
- Severe pain is present.
- Excessive drooling is present in a child older than 1 year of age who looks very ill, especially if un-immunized.
- One tonsil appears markedly larger than the other.
- There is a marked redness or rapid swelling of lymph nodes visible on the outside of the neck.
- There is progressive lethargy, irritability, or fever greater than 105 degrees.
- Your child has any difficulty breathing.
- Your child is not able to open his mouth wide without severe pain.
- Your child has a recent history of falling with a sharp object in his mouth.
- Your child develops stridor that cannot be controlled by measures listed in this handbook under the "Croup" section.
- Your child develops blood in the urine or brown urine.

Call within 24 hours if:
- Your child has a sore throat and has been exposed to strep.
- The sore throat persists longer than 7 days.
- There is increased difficulty swallowing or breathing.

- Any rash develops, especially a sunburned-looking, sandpaper-feeling rash during the illness.
- Hives develop along with the sore throat.
- Fever lasts more than 5 days.
- The sore throat causes dehydration. (Your infant/toddler has not urinated in the last 8 hours, or your child older than 2 years has not urinated in more than 12 hours.) See "Dehydration" section.
- Your child has recently recovered from strep and develops strep-like symptoms again within only a few days or weeks after antibiotic treatment.
- A lymph node in the neck becomes extremely large.
- Abdominal pain is increasingly uncomfortable.

 ## Other Relevant Sections

Bronchiolitis

Bronchitis

Colds

Croup

Earache/Ear Infection

Fever

Hives

Infectious Mononucleosis

Influenza

Lymph Nodes

Sinus Infection

Integrated Management of Respiratory Illnesses

 ## Prevention

Prevention should be focused on the causative agent. For example, if a dry climate is the culprit, a humidifier should be used. If allergies are suspected, identification of the triggering agent, avoidance of it, and treatment of allergy symptoms are recommended.

For viral infections and bacterial infections, the infectious agents are transmitted through the air as well as in contaminated oral and nasal secretions. As always, careful hand-washing is the key. Caregivers and the child should be meticulous in washing hands and objects touched by the ill child. Discourage the sharing of eating utensils and drinks with each other. Infectious sore throats can be passed on to another person up to 24 hours before the symptoms even begin. Teach your children to keep their hands away from their nose, eyes, and mouth as much as possible, and to cover the nose and mouth when sneezing and coughing.

Avoid children known to be ill either with strep or viral sore throats. Avoid contact with cigarette smoke and other environmental irritants. You might also get a new toothbrush for your child.

Never allow your young child to walk around with utensils, sticks, or other similar objects in his mouth.

Description/Physiology

Thrush is a common problem seen primarily in infancy and rarely seen after 1 year of age. It is characterized by white patches that coat the insides of the cheeks and sometimes the tongue. On occasion, the gums and lips may be involved. These filmy patches cannot easily be wiped off.

Thrush is caused by an overgrowth of yeast, which lives normally in the mouth. Certain triggers cause yeast overgrowth and this creates the visible patches of white. Beneath the white film is inflamed tissue.

Most children will never develop thrush, while a small percentage will and may even have several recurrent bouts during the first year. Ultimately, all children outgrow this tendency.

 ## Causes/Epidemiology

Thrush is caused by a yeast called Candida albicans, which grows naturally on the lining of the mouth. Normally, the yeast lives in harmony with other organisms and enzymes in the mouth unless there is a trigger that disturbs the balance. When that happens, the yeast concentration increases, so much so that the colonies gather into the white patches you see.

Several triggers may disrupt this delicate balance: prolonged sucking; additional yeast colonization from mother's infected nipples; antibiotics taken by a breast-feeding mother, which are passed into the breast milk and on to the baby; or antibiotics that the baby may take directly for a bacterial infection. An antibiotic disrupts the balance between oral yeast and oral bacteria because the mouth bacteria normally keep the growth of yeast at bay. When the antibiotic kills certain mouth bacteria, yeast tends to overgrow in greater amounts than the body can handle by itself.

 ## Expected Course

Thrush develops slowly over a period of a few days. Initially, it may be mistaken for breast milk or formula that remains on the tongue or cheeks after feeds. Eventually, however, it becomes clear that this is a white film adherent to the tongue and cheeks and cannot be easily wiped off. It is usually mild and does not typically interfere with feeding or sleep. Otherwise, there are usually no other symptoms associated with thrush.

THRUSH (ORAL YEAST INFECTION)

On occasion, thrush can be quite advanced, with a very thick white coat and cheesy-looking patches with considerable inflammation underneath. These children may have a disruption in their feeding because of discomfort with sucking. Advanced thrush may also interfere with sleep.

The majority of infants with thrush respond to treatment well (see below). There are some, however, who do not clear easily and may require lengthy treatment.

There are very few complications with thrush. Some infants may also develop a simultaneous yeast diaper rash. See the "Diaper Rash" section. In very rare instances, a child may refuse to eat and become mildly dehydrated. Please see "Dehydration" section.

 ## Contagiousness/Immunity

Thrush is rarely contagious from one child to another. However, the yeast may be transmitted to mother's nipple by breast-feeding. Because of the abrading nature of the baby's suck, mother's nipple may be infected by the baby's oral yeast. Mothers report red, cracked, and even bleeding nipples. Nipples can be very tender, itchy, flaky, and burning. The pain can be intense with breast-feeding and make feeding quite difficult.

 ## Home Care

The goals of home care are to restore the natural balance of the mouth by eliminating yeast overgrowth and to provide relief for mother and infant.

We ask you to first read through the entire "Home Care" section to select those recommendations which make the most sense in your child's situation.

1. Anti-yeast medication. Prescription medications are usually provided for treating thrush. The most common treatment is called Nystatin oral suspension. Your prescription will direct you to place 1 to 2 cc inside each cheek and on the tongue about 15 minutes after each meal. This may mean that you administer the medication 6 to 8 times per day. This is perfectly safe.

   If the thrush is not improving after 4 to 5 days, you may gently rub the Nystatin directly onto the affected areas with a cotton swab. In most cases, the thrush will improve within 5 to 7 days. Treat until all the thrush has disappeared and continue for 3 additional days.

   If you are breast-feeding, apply Nystatin cream to your irritated nipples at least twice daily. Be sure to gently rinse the Nystatin cream from your nipples prior to breast-feeding. If the thrush returns, you may follow the same procedure.

If the Nystatin does not work after 10 days, your health-care provider may prescribe another oral medication.

2. Decrease sucking time. If eating and sucking are painful for your child or you have extreme pain with breast-feeding, try using a bottle temporarily. A syringe or cup may also be necessary. The key here is to reduce sucking time to 10 to 15 minutes per feeding.

3. Pacifier use. Be sure the pacifier has been cleaned regularly, usually by running it through the dishwasher or immersing it in boiling water for 2 to 3 minutes. You may want to replace the pacifier during the treatment of thrush, to help prevent recurrence.

4. Diaper rash. If your child has an associated diaper rash, it is safe to assume it is also due to yeast. You should try an anti-fungal cream, such as Lotrimin®AF on the rash. See "Diaper Rash" section.

5. Discomfort. The inflammation that underlies thrush may cause irritability, which further disrupts sleep. You may try acetaminophen and see if that relieves the discomfort. See "OTC Medication Recommendations and Dosages" section. Infants less than 2 months of age and with fever greater than 100 degrees (rectal) must be brought to your health-care provider's attention right away.

6. Patch management. Do not try to scrape off or pick away the patches of thrush. This will only serve to create more inflammation and pain.

 ## Integrated Therapies

(Please refer to the section on "Administering Integrated Treatments" on page 19 for guidance on using any of the therapies that follow.)

HERBAL REMEDIES (For quick reference please refer to the "Herbal Remedies List" on page 31 and the inside cover.)

• Aloe vera gel (food grade) may be swabbed with a cotton swab directly onto the thrush up to 3 times a day.

HOMEOPATHIC REMEDIES (For quick reference please refer to the "Homeopathic Remedies List" on page 32 and the inside cover.)

• A homeopathic remedy designed to decrease inflammation and fever from infections may help prevent deterioration and improve the recovery time. It can be taken 3 to 6 times daily until the thrush is cleared. (General Support 2)

- A homeopathic remedy designed to speed the body's recovery from inflammation may help to minimize swelling and inflammation. It may be taken (1 tablet or 4 drops per dose) 3 to 6 times a day until the thrush is healed. (General Support 4)

NUTRITIONALS AND SUPPLEMENTS

- Acidophilus (baby-specific product), especially if mother received antibiotics during the pregnancy or while breast-feeding or the infant has received antibiotics. For infants, we generally suggest that you mix the recommended dose with a small amount of breast milk or formula and gently syringe it into his mouth twice a day until the thrush has resolved.

 When to Call Your Health-care Provider

Thrush is not an emergency, and all calls can safely be made the following morning.

Call within 24 hours if:
- Your child refuses to nurse or bottle-feed.
- The thrush worsens once treatment has begun.
- The thrush lasts beyond 14 days, even with treatment.

 Other Relevant Sections

Diaper Rash

 Prevention

Aggressive prevention is rarely needed. For children with recurrent thrush, techniques such as limiting pacifier time and cleansing the pacifier are helpful. In addition, careful breast hygiene will reduce the risk of repeated thrush. For example, avoid long stretches when the nipples remain moist. Allow them to air-dry often during the day.

Description/Physiology

Urinary tract infections (UTIs) are bacterial infections that may involve some or all of the structures of the urinary tract: the kidneys, the ureter (the tube that connects the kidneys with the bladder), the bladder, and the urethra (the tube that connects the bladder with the outside of the body). UTIs are relatively common in children, especially in young girls and adolescent women. They are much less common in boys.

A urinary tract infection may present with pain, burning with urination, increased frequency of urination, abdominal pain, fever, blood in the urine, incontinence (urinary accidents), back pain, diarrhea, and vomiting.

A UTI is nearly always a bacterial infection. Urine itself is sterile (bacteria-free) in normal health and can become colonized by bacteria in one of three ways. The most common mechanism is migration of bacteria up the urethra and into the bladder. This process is accelerated by any event that increases urinary retention or incomplete voiding, such as burning pain from vaginitis or urethritis. In girls, the urethra is much shorter than in boys and is located close to areas with significant bacterial colonization such as the vagina and rectum. Therefore, the frequency of a UTI is much greater in girls than in boys.

Secondly, bacteria may also be carried from another site of infection through the bloodstream and then invade the urinary system. This is a very uncommon mechanism in otherwise healthy children.

Finally, bacteria may enter the urinary system directly from an infection in an adjacent structure right next to the kidneys or bladder. This is also an uncommon mechanism.

Once the bacteria have colonized the urine, they may multiply rapidly, resulting in an infection. Shortly thereafter, the child may become symptomatic.

In little girls, a condition called vaginitis (inflammation of the vagina), and in little boys, a condition called urethritis (inflammation of the urethra), can both begin with symptoms like a UTI in its early stages. Generally, an irritant such as soap, bubble bath, shampoo, stool, sand, or dried urine (especially in the older, non-toilet-trained children or bed-wetters) inflames the linings of the genitals and causes pain and discomfort with urination. The discomfort of a urinary tract infection is usually more severe than that of vaginitis or urethritis. However, all three may present with a screaming child, holding her bottom, and refusing to urinate. Vaginitis is far more common than a urinary tract infection. The pain associated with vaginitis and/or urethritis can predispose a child to developing a UTI because of the urinary retention they cause.

URINARY TRACT INFECTION

 ## Causes/Epidemiology

The majority of UTIs are bacterial, most commonly E. coli. There is a clear prevalence in girls over boys. On rare occasions, a virus may infect the urinary tract and will usually be localized to the bladder. In some cases, a viral cystitis (bladder infection) can lead to visible blood in the urine.

Poor wiping techniques, constipation, malnutrition, diabetes, urine retention, and in adolescents, sexual intercourse, may also trigger a UTI. There is a slightly higher risk of UTIs in uncircumcised males. On occasion, tight irritating or constrictive clothing can lead to a UTI.

Trauma to this area, especially to the urethra, may also produce symptoms like a UTI, including pain and blood in the urine.

 ## Expected Course

The course of a UTI depends on the age of the child, the method by which it was triggered, and the general health of the child. In most cases, when bacteria reach part of the urinary system where they do not belong, the body's own natural immune system will repel the invading bacteria. For example, the force of the urine stream alone may wash the invading bacteria out of the urethra, and the lining of the bladder also resists bacterial growth. If sufficient bacterial colonies grow, they can overcome the body's defenses and multiply rapidly, and symptoms will begin to develop.

In infants, symptoms may be non-specific, such as irritability, low-grade fever, and poor feeding. There may be a foul or bitter smell to the urine. These symptoms may continue for a number of days and be assumed to be a viral illness. Eventually, though, infants and toddlers with a UTI will develop a fever, more irritability, blood in the diaper, complete loss of appetite, vomiting, dehydration, and even show specific signs of urinary pain. A physical examination is not likely to reveal a source of the infection, but a urine sample for analysis and culture will reveal the presence of a UTI.

Most infants respond well to antibiotic therapy. If a recurrent pattern of UTIs emerges, additional testing will be needed. In boys, UTIs are uncommon and may occur because of an underlying anatomical abnormality of the urinary system. Therefore, boys with a first UTI will warrant immediate investigation.

Older children with a UTI may complain of pain with urination, itching, increased urinary frequency including the inability to make it through the night without urination, and fever. The urine may be dark and foul-smelling. The child may also be lethargic and complain of stomachache or backache. Toilet-trained children may become incontinent. Abdominal pain, irritability, lethargy, and restless sleep may also be seen. As the infection progresses, the child may develop more exaggerated symptoms, with blood in the urine, refusal to urinate, vomiting, or even dehydration.

If only the bladder is involved (cystitis), the UTI tends to be milder. If the kidneys and ureter are involved, the infection will have a more significant impact. Kidney infections (pyelonephritis) are usually more serious infections and may require IV antibiotics, IV hydration, and hospitalization. These children are often quite toxic and may present with a very high fever (greater than 104 degrees), abdominal pain, vomiting, severe back pain, chills, and lethargy. A bladder infection may trigger "reflux" of infected urine up the ureter to ultimately reach the kidney. It may also be the case that the reflux is already present and the UTI makes it worse. Even severe pyelonephritis generally responds well to treatment.

Several other illnesses may appear very similar to a UTI. A bad case of the flu, viral gastroenteritis, and even diabetes may all behave similar to UTIs. Diabetes may present with more frequent urination but is also accompanied by excessive thirst, hunger, and often with fatigue and weight loss. Generally, specific symptoms related to the urinary tract point us toward a UTI diagnosis.

A urinalysis and a urine culture are essential to the diagnosis of a UTI. Your health-care provider may send a urine sample for bacterial culture. The urine is cultured for 48 hours to identify the specific bacteria responsible for the infection and to determine the best antibiotic for treatment.

After antibiotic treatment, the urine must be re-cultured. Should the infection persist, another antibiotic may be recommended. A radiologic study of the urinary tract and/or an evaluation of the urinary system by a urologist may be recommended.

 ## Contagiousness/Immunity

UTIs are not contagious. It is essentially impossible to transmit the bacteria of one child's UTI to another child's urinary system. Even viral cystitis triggers are rarely transmitted between children.

URINARY TRACT INFECTION

🏠 Home Care

If your child has a more superficial infection (for example, urethritis or vaginitis), home care will probably relieve symptoms with minimal treatment. If a more advanced infection exists (cystitis or pyelonephritis), more aggressive therapy will be required. In these situations your health-care provider may start an antibiotic pre-emptively, pending the confirmation by urine culture.

The goals for home care overlap with office-care goals. Once the diagnosis of a bacterial urinary tract infection is established, an antibiotic will be prescribed or continued. In the meantime, home care should focus on pain relief, preservation of hydration, and general comforting measures.

We ask you to first read the entire "Home Care" section and select those treatments that make the most sense given your child's situation.

1. First, try sitz baths in warm, clear water. Place your child in the tub (girls should be in a squatting position to increase genital exposure to the rinsing water). Bathe him/her 5 to 10 minutes, 2 to 3 times per day in water as warm as can be tolerated. Children who refuse to urinate due to pain may be encouraged to urinate directly into the bathwater as this will reduce the pain.

2. Encourage your child to drink lots of fluids to better flush the urinary system and to decrease lengthy bladder retention of urine.

3 Use Lotrimin® cream to protect irritated labia or skin around genitals from the risk of yeast overgrowth, especially if there is an accompanying diaper rash or labial irritation. Apply it to any irritated area after every sitz bath.

4. Use acetaminophen or ibuprofen for fever discomfort and pain relief. See "OTC Medication Recommendations and Dosages" section. In general, ibuprofen is a more effective pain reliever.

5. If your child has a cystitis or pyelonephritis, once the diagnosis has been established, your health-care provider may prescribe or continue an antibiotic. If your child shows no signs of improvement within 2 to 3 days, or is getting worse even on antibiotics, call your health-care provider.

6. Avoid acidic foods such as citrus fruits.

Integrated Therapies

(Please refer to the section on "Administering Integrated Treatments" on page 19 for guidance on using any of the therapies that follow.)

HERBAL REMEDIES (For quick reference please refer to the "Herbal Remedies List" on page 31 and the inside cover.)

- Valerian root is a mild herbal sedative that may offer some help in easing a child with significant restlessness or pain. Valerian root may be most useful at bedtime. For dosing, follow the package labeling accurately.
- Cranberry can be very effective in helping to resolve inflammation in the urinary tract. Cranberry juices, if consumed in large enough amounts, can be effective. Cranberry can also be found as a capsule, chewable tablet, or liquid concentrate, which is probably a more effective method of delivery. For dosing, follow the package labeling accurately.

HOMEOPATHIC REMEDIES (For quick reference please refer to the "Homeopathic Remedies List" on page 32 and the inside cover.)

- A homeopathic remedy designed to decrease inflammation and fever from infections may help prevent deterioration and improve the recovery time. It can be taken 3 to 6 times daily when the virus is active (for example, fever, lethargy, etc.). (General Support 2)
- A homeopathic remedy designed to restore balance to bladder function may help to prevent deterioration and improve the recovery time. It can be taken 2 to 3 times daily during the illness. (Urinary 1)

BACH FLOWER REMEDIES

- Rescue Remedy™ may be of use if your child is uncomfortable from the illness, stress, or anxiety. You may use 2 drops every 10 minutes to every few hours to calm restlessness as needed.
- A lukewarm bath with 10 drops of Rescue Remedy™ added to the bathwater is often very effective at relieving agitation and stress in general.

NUTRITIONALS AND SUPPLEMENTS

- Vitamin C
- Probiotics are especially important if your child is put on an antibiotic.

URINARY TRACT INFECTION

DIETARY GUIDELINES

- If your child enjoys cranberry juice (either by itself or as a mixed juice), he/she may drink liberal quantities during the treatment.
- Your child may not feel well enough to eat, so don't force it. Instead, make sure that there is a good intake of fluids and extra water to ensure good hydration. You may use the following table as a general guideline for water in addition to normal fluid intake:

AGE	OUNCES OF WATER PER DAY
2 to 5 years old	12 to 18 ounces
5 to 12 years old	18 to 24 ounces
13 and up	32 to 48 ounces

 When to Call Your Health-care Provider

Call immediately if any of the following occur:

- Pain is worsening rapidly.
- Your child starts acting very ill.
- Your child develops a fever that exceeds 104 degrees.
- Your child cannot urinate, even during or after sitz baths.
- Bloody, cloudy, or foul-smelling urine develops.
- Your child develops significant back pain and abdominal pain.
- Your child begins to vomit repeatedly and is at risk for dehydration. See "Dehydration" section.

Call within 24 hours if:

- Symptoms are no better in 48 to 72 hours after the above measures have been tried.
- Abdominal pain or back pain progresses.
- Over time, your child becomes more lethargic and uncomfortable.
- A rash appears after antibiotics are started.
- Your child is having more frequent urinary accidents, or new bedwetting symptoms.
- Your child is developing more frequent urination, excessive thirst, and increased appetite.

Other Relevant Sections

Abdominal Pain

Constipation

Dehydration

Diaper Rash

Fever

 ## Prevention

Avoid bubble bath. The bathwater should be absolutely clear—no shampoo, bubble bath, or floating soap bars during the playtime part of the bath. The genitals should be gently rinsed with clear water at the end of the bath to remove any remaining soap residue that may linger in the delicate tissue folds. You may even encourage your child to urinate during the bath. Cotton underwear is best.

Always wipe stool from front to back in young girls. Prevent your child from becoming constipated. See "Constipation" section. Chronic constipation may be a trigger for UTIs. Encourage your child to urinate at least every 3 to 4 hours during the day and to "not hold it in." This allows the frequent flushing of the urethra to prevent the bacteria from migrating up into the bladder. Drinking lots of water will help maintain good urine flow.

GENERAL INFORMATION

Most children who receive vaccines experience no reactions at all, or very mild reactions such as fever or soreness at the site of injection. Very rarely, allergic or more severe reactions may occur, but statistically, being vaccinated is still far safer than contracting the diseases that the vaccines prevent.

Your child should not receive a vaccine if he:

- Is ill with a fever greater than 100 degrees within 24 hours of the visit.
- Has a documented allergy to a vaccine component (for example, eggs with the MMR vaccine).
- Has experienced a severe reaction to a past vaccine of that same type, for example:
  - inconsolable crying for 3 hours or more
  - a fever of 105 degrees or more
  - seizure
  - limp, pale, and/or dusky spells
  - an unusual high-pitched cry with lethargy

If your child experiences a severe reaction or if you have concerns about his reaction to a vaccine, notify your health-care provider.

Rarely, a child may experience a serious anaphylactic, allergic reaction to a vaccine. Symptoms of allergic reactions include wheezing, hoarseness, and difficulty breathing. Should these symptoms develop, seek immediate medical attention or call 911.

COMMON "ACCEPTABLE" REACTIONS AND HOME CARE TREATMENT

1. Mild fever (100 to 103 degrees) in the 48 hours following immunization is common and can be treated with acetaminophen or ibuprofen (see "OTC Medication Recommendations and Dosages" section). There is no evidence that severe reactions can be prevented in this manner.

2. Many children also experience mild pain, tenderness, warmth, and swelling at the site of the injection. Cool compresses and the use of acetaminophen or ibuprofen can help treat pain or swelling. Please see "OTC Medication Recommendations and Dosages" section.

3. Elevation of the head when sleeping may help minimize headache. NOTE: Do not use pillows for children less than 2 years of age.

4. Sometimes a small nodule (a hard lump) will form in the thigh at the injection site. This may take several days to weeks to completely resolve.

5. Following the Varicella (chickenpox) vaccine a rash may develop at the injection site. This should resolve in a few days but may spread chickenpox to others who have not had chickenpox if there is skin-to-skin contact. For that reason, keep the rash covered until it resolves.

6. Following the MMR vaccine your child may develop swelling of lymph nodes in the neck and/or under the jaw. This will usually resolve in a few days and only requires observation. Mild joint pain or stiffness may be noted in the first 48 hours and at 10 to 14 days after the shot. This will usually resolve within a few days.

7. The INFLUENZA (injectable) vaccine is a "killed" virus vaccine; one cannot get the flu from the vaccine itself. It is not uncommon, however, for children to experience mild side effects such as fever (usually less than 103 degrees), soreness, redness, or swelling at the vaccine site, aches, and mild exhaustion or fatigue. These symptoms begin soon after the shot and usually last only 1 to 2 days.

 ## When to Call Your Health-care Provider

Call if:
- Allergic or serious reaction is suspected (see above).
- The area of redness and tenderness at shot site becomes progressively worse over 48 hours, rather than gradually improving.
- Your child has a seizure, difficulty breathing, dusky/blue color change (call 911 if child is unstable).
- Your child develops progressive weakness of the extremity days after the shot.

The most up-to-date information on these and any other vaccines can be found at www.cdc.gov/nip/vacsafe or at www.aap.org.

VOMITING

 Description/Physiology

Vomiting is one of the most common symptoms in childhood. It can occur in any age group. Vomiting is defined as the forceful expulsion of stomach contents through the mouth. This is in contrast to regurgitation or spitting up (very common in young infants), in which formula or breast milk are ejected less forcefully in an otherwise well-appearing infant.

To begin with, a bit of descriptive anatomy may be helpful. When food or saliva are swallowed, they first pass into the esophagus (food pipe), and enter the stomach by passing through a sphincter called the lower esophageal sphincter (LES). The LES acts as a one-way valve, which protects the esophagus from the backward movement (reflux or vomiting) of stomach contents. The stomach itself lies across the top of the abdomen, roughly at the level of the lower central margin of the rib cage. It is a sac that stretches easily to accommodate food, and it produces acids and enzymes used in digestion. At the end of the stomach is another valve, called the pylorus, which leads into the first part of the intestine, the duodenum.

The stomach is one of the first sites of digestion. Tremendous amounts of acid are produced there to begin this process. Regardless of its cause, vomiting is triggered by the involuntary contraction of the smooth muscle of the stomach lining, which sweeps its contents upward, along the path of least resistance, back through the lower esophageal sphincter (LES), up through the esophagus, then into and out of the mouth.

 Causes/Epidemiology

There are many causes of vomiting in children. It is impossible to discuss each cause in depth in this handbook, but we will highlight the most common triggers. Causes are influenced by the age of the child, his own general health, and the child's anatomy.

In infants, the most common cause is simply "spitting up," which is nothing more than the passive movement of stomach contents, usually after a feeding, back up the esophagus. This may be because your baby has been overfed, has a weak LES, is in a horizontal (lying down flat) position after a meal, has swallowed too much air, and/or is developing a virus.

Most spitting up in babies is benign and rarely leads to problems such as dehydration. In fact, most "spitty" babies thrive, are smiling and happy, and seem unaffected by the spitting.

308

Other infants, however, may manage a strong vomit with some wretching that is clearly more than spitting up. There may even be a projectile arc to the vomiting. Again, this is usually benign and triggered by one or more of the factors listed above. One or two episodes like this a day is common in newborns and infants.

However, we worry when the frequency of vomiting, especially projectile, increases. In newborns as young as 1 to 2 weeks, if this progressive pattern develops, and especially if the child is a firstborn male, we would be concerned about a disease called pyloric stenosis. Pyloric stenosis is characterized by the muscular tightening of the end portion of the stomach (the pylorus). The pylorus is squeezed so tightly that stomach contents cannot easily pass through it into the first part of the intestine and thus are projected back up the esophagus. This is a congenital problem and there is often a family history. The diagnosis usually requires a radiological study and the treatment is most often a surgical repair.

Other infants who present with frequent vomiting, especially with arching and pain, may have gastro-esophageal reflux disease (GERD). This is an extremely common problem in infants and thought to be a major contributor to colic. See "Colic" section. In these cases, however, children do not generally projectile vomit in the same fashion as with pyloric stenosis and are rarely dehydrated. But reflux may persist for several months until the LES has become a fully functional valve which keeps stomach contents where they belong. Reflux and colic respond to many of the same treatment measures as described below.

In toddlers and children, one of the most common causes of vomiting is a viral infection. There are many different gastrointestinal viruses that can cause the "stomach flu" with vomiting. These viruses occur throughout the year but are especially prevalent in the warmer months. For example, rotavirus is one such virus.

Bacterial infections may also cause vomiting. Common examples include salmonella, shigella, E.coli, and staph. Food poisoning is often bacterial and almost always causes vomiting. Children with strep or a urinary tract infection may also have vomiting.

A parasitic infection called giardia can be contracted through exposure to contaminated water and in daycare settings, where giardia is easily transmitted. Giardia is often contracted in the mountains and during travel.

Almost any illness that is severe or any organ system that is significantly impaired may trigger a defensive response to that illness and produce vomiting. Other causes of vomiting include head trauma, forceful coughing, reactions to medications, allergies or intolerance to certain foods, pain, and trauma in general. Motion sickness, constipation, muscle strain, exhaustion, emotional upset, anxiety, and fear are other triggers. Mild causes such as teething or excessive crying can cause a susceptible child to vomit.

Any obstruction or blockage at some point in the gastro-intestinal system may cause vomiting. Pyloric stenosis is just one such example, but there are several points along the GI tract where a blockage may occur. Obstruction is much less common in children, although children with a history of abdominal surgery are more susceptible.

Appendicitis may also present with vomiting. The classic symptoms include pain onset around the belly button, with a shift of pain to the right lower quadrant of the abdomen; loss of appetite; low-grade fever; nausea; vomiting; and diarrhea. The progression of pain is usually focused in the right lower quadrant and is the strongest indication that your child may have appendicitis.

There may have been recent injury directly to the abdomen, which may produce acute vomiting as well as later onset vomiting. For example, a handlebar injury to the abdomen could injure the stomach or other important abdominal organs such as the liver, spleen, or pancreas.

It is also possible that your child could have swallowed a foreign object that may be sharp or too large to pass out of the stomach.

Some adolescents vomit voluntarily, as with bulimia. Others may vomit after drug or alcohol ingestion. In rare instances, vomiting may be due to morning sickness associated with pregnancy.

Your careful history and observations and your health-care provider's physical examination will give the best information for the correct diagnosis. On occasion, lab testing will help make that determination.

 ## Expected Course

The course of a vomiting disorder depends on the age of the child, the trigger for the vomiting, and the severity of associated symptoms.

Infants typically regurgitate intermittently in the first few months of life. In addition, there are those babies who consistently vomit once or twice a day. In most cases, even these babies gain weight, thrive, and grow normally. The few interventions needed as described below may help these babies until they outgrow this tendency.

For babies with severe reflux and vomiting, several measures may need to be used to bring relief and ensure good growth. These babies develop vomiting and colic-like symptoms within one or two weeks of birth, and they may present with classic irritability, frequent spitting or vomiting, and tightening of the abdomen.

Babies with symptoms of colic may have gurgly stomachs, draw up their legs, and pass gas. See "Colic" section. Not all colic is the result of reflux, nor is all vomiting in infants related to reflux. But many of the colic-relieving measures may help an infant who is prone to vomiting.

For infants with pyloric stenosis, vomiting is so severe that the child may become dehydrated. Vomiting may occur after every feeding and with increasing force and frequency. This diagnosis is made either through ultrasound or an X-ray. If the diagnosis is confirmed, a surgeon will be consulted to evaluate and correct the problem.

Vomiting from viruses is usually short-lived (12 to 36 hours) and improves with measures stated below. Abdominal pain, diarrhea, nausea, and fever often accompany these vomiting episodes. In some cases, the vomiting and general symptoms may be so severe (especially in the presence of diarrhea) that dehydration may occur. See "Dehydration" section.

In bacterial illnesses with vomiting, the symptoms may be more severe than with viral triggers. These children often have diarrhea, nausea, frequent vomiting, fever, lethargy, malaise, and abdominal pain. Bloody diarrhea is a frequent accompanying symptom. These children, too, are at risk for dehydration.

With bacterial food poisoning, the onset of vomiting is usually abrupt. A child will experience rapid onset of nausea, early abdominal cramping, and vomiting. The child may vomit repeatedly, be doubled over in pain, and have a fever, chills, sweats, and extreme agitation. The vomiting may also stop fairly abruptly, although the child may continue to be weak and have some abdominal pain and nausea. Most children with food poisoning can be managed at home, but occasionally the vomiting is so severe that a visit to your health-care provider or the ER will be warranted for evaluation, IV hydration, and even hospitalization.

Children with giardia may also have vomiting, abdominal pain, abdominal distension, flatulence, diarrhea, and low-grade fever. These symptoms may be mild and persist for several weeks before a diagnosis is made. There may also be blood in the stool. Giardia may also produce a more severe illness with significant diarrhea and abdominal pain.

Children with head trauma may vomit once or twice as a natural reaction to the stress of the injury. Repeated vomiting causes greater concern that there may be a skull fracture, brain injury, or concussion. Please see the "Head Injury" section.

Children who cough forcibly may trigger vomiting called "post-tussive emesis." This vomiting will lessen when the cough is controlled. This vomiting is often caused by swallowed mucous, some nausea, and the sheer force of the cough triggering a "gag reflex."

Food intolerance or an "allergic reaction" to a food may cause vomiting. You may observe this as you introduce new solid foods. If you suspect food intolerance, it is best to discuss this with your health-care provider.

A discussion of bulimia is beyond the scope of this book. If you suspect your child has bulimia, please call your health-care provider ASAP.

Some complications are common with vomiting, again depending on the triggering event. Vomiting blood may result from torn blood vessels in the esophagus or stomach lining, ulcers, or from swallowed foreign bodies. Dehydration remains the most common complication.

 ## Contagiousness/Immunity

All viral causes for vomiting are contagious. They are transmitted through oral secretions, vomitus and stool contamination, passed from one child or adult to another. This is also true of giardia.

Most bacterial infections are transmitted through improperly stored or prepared food. Undercooked meat and potato salads at picnics are frequent culprits.

Most infectious illnesses are no longer contagious when the fever (if present) has disappeared and the gastro-intestinal symptoms, whether vomiting or diarrhea, have improved substantially. It is impossible to know the exact moment at which your child is no longer contagious. For school and daycare purposes, we recommend that your child no longer has fever, vomiting, or diarrhea for approximately 48 hours before returning to school or daycare. Many daycares ask that diarrhea volume subside enough to be contained within a diaper. Please consult your daycare provider.

Other causes of vomiting, such as obstruction, food intolerance, and reflux, are, of course, not contagious.

 ## Home Care

The treatment of vomiting depends on the primary cause of vomiting, the age of the child, the presence of other symptoms, and the presence of dehydration.

Although vomiting can be frightening, it is rarely an emergency. The vast majority of vomiting can be controlled by the measures listed below.

To help you assess the severity of the vomiting and dehydration, here are several questions to ask yourself and observations to make. In addition, it is a good idea to begin to record this information in a log to create accurate documentation of the illness.

In your log note the following:

- The number of vomiting episodes.
- The type of vomiting—for example, projectile, minimal force, spitting up.
- Other associated symptoms, especially fever, lethargy, irritability, nausea.
- The number of diarrhea episodes present (if any).
- How often your child is urinating.
- Any other family members with a similar illness?
- Has your child had similar episodes in the past?

This type of information will be helpful for your health-care provider to assess the severity of the disease, to make the correct diagnosis, and to recommend its subsequent treatment.

The primary goals for treatment of vomiting are to provide comfort, prevent dehydration, and support your child's own immune system until the cause has been eliminated and balance restored.

Every child is different, and we cannot make exact recommendations for every unique vomiting situation; however, the principles below will generally manage the vast majority of vomiting children. We encourage you to read through the entire "Home Care" section first before you do anything to identify which recommendations make the most sense for your child's particular situation.

1. Stop all oral intake (liquids and solids) for at least 1 to 2 hours. If you can comfort your child to sleep, this sleep will provide a natural pause in drinking that may allow the body to "regroup." This time will also allow the stomach to empty its current contents. An infant of less than 6 months, of course, will need fluids within 1 to 2 hours, so they require special attention and treatment. For infants, a short period of stopping breast-feeding or formula-feeding is advised. In the early part of the illness, an older child may manage 6 to 8 hours without fluid intake.

2. After this period of stomach rest, begin with clear liquids. In infants, oral electrolyte solutions, such as Pedialyte® (use unflavored for infants under 6 months of age), are best. If this is refused, you may offer diluted pumped breast milk with water, or, if formula-fed, diluted formula with water. Dilutions should begin with 1 ounce of formula or breast milk to 3 ounces of water.

   For breast-fed babies who refuse to take a bottle, you might first start feeding with only one breast. If vomiting continues, try limiting the time at that one breast to less than 10 minutes.

   In older babies or toddlers, you may also try Pedialyte® (flavored or unflavored). If this is refused, you may need to try 1/2 strength

VOMITING

Gatorade®, very flat soda pop (especially "de-fizzed" ginger ale, lemon-lime, or cola), warm herbal teas, or water itself. Popsicles may be useful as they provide a slow trickle of fluids.

3. Begin very slowly by giving ½ to 1 ounce of liquid every 20 minutes for 1 to 2 hours while your child is awake. If this small amount is held down, advance to 1 to 2 ounces of clear liquids every 30 to 60 minutes for several more hours. Do not continue clear liquids only, without solids, for longer than 24 hours without calling your health-care provider. Infants may tolerate only 1 teaspoonful of liquid at first, but you can gradually build volume to 1 to 2 ounces. If an infant or child vomits at any point in this slow advance of fluids, give him another rest period of 30 to 60 minutes and try again at the point where you left off, or you may try offering 1 to 2 teaspoons every 5 to 10 minutes, gradually increasing the volume.

4. Do not give cold liquids. Room-temperature fluids are always better tolerated.

5. Your child may want larger amounts of liquid or even desire solids. Resist the temptation to give larger volumes of fluid or solids until he has gone 4 to 6 hours without vomiting, as the distension of the stomach could trigger vomiting. A gradual build-up of volume will help preserve what has already been drunk. Use your best judgment, but, in general, it is always best to go very slowly when increasing volumes.

6. If the above measures do not work, you should stop all oral intake again for another hour or so. Once the vomiting has stopped, begin the use of Emetrol®, an over-the-counter medication for vomiting, in a dose of 1 to 2 teaspoons every 20 minutes for 1 hour. If Emetrol® is retained, give 1 teaspoon of Emetrol® once every hour along with clear liquids as directed above. Emetrol® acts as a mild "buffer" of the stomach's acidity and helps reduce stomach contractions.

7. After 12 to 24 hours of no vomiting, your child may very gradually return to a normal diet. Begin first with bland solids: applesauce, cereals without milk, bananas, dry toast, crackers, and mashed potatoes. Dairy products should be avoided for 3 to 5 days in older children.

   Formula in smaller infants should first be reintroduced at half-strength concentration for 1 to 2 days, then on to full-strength after that. Breast-fed infants should resume feeding with short, but more frequent feedings. The original breast-feeding routine can be reintroduced within 12 to 24 hours after vomiting has stopped.

8. Discontinue all medicines for 6 to 8 hours. Also stop antibiotics for 6 to 8 hours, and if the vomiting has stopped, you may try the antibiotic again. If the antibiotic is vomited, hold off until the next day. If it is again vomited, call your health-care provider. You may want to mix the antibiotic with a bit of Pedialyte® or water to reduce the concentration. Oral medicines may irritate the stomach and worsen vomiting. If your child needs fever relief, use acetaminophen rectal suppositories. See "OTC Medication Recommendations and Dosages" section. Call your health-care provider if your child needs to continue taking a prescription medicine (for example, for seizures or asthma) but is vomiting.

9. In general, there is no effective and safe "drug therapy" or suppository for vomiting. Anti-vomiting suppositories, by prescription, may be used on occasion after your health-care provider has assessed the cause of the vomiting and your child's degree of hydration. They are rarely necessary in children, because the vomiting is usually self-limited, and when it is not, IV hydration (which often stops the vomiting) is frequently required.

10. Keep the head of the bed or crib positioned at an angle. Keep your child upright for at least 30 minutes after each feeding or drinking.

Integrated Therapies

(Please refer to the section on "Administering Integrated Treatments" on page 19 for guidance on using any of the therapies that follow.)

AROMATHERAPY

- An aromatherapy bath or massage with the essential oils of eucalyptus radiata and/or lavender can soothe and relax your child's anxiety and restlessness. Add 2 to 5 drops of oil to a warm bath and allow your child to soak for a comfortable period of time.

HERBAL REMEDIES (For quick reference please refer to the "Herbal Remedies List" on page 31 and the inside cover.)

- Ginger is a valuable herb that may be helpful to quiet down an "upset stomach," decrease abdominal cramping, and soothe nausea. It may be useful until the vomiting subsides. For dosing, follow the package labeling accurately.
- Mint can also soothe an upset stomach. Mint teas, lightly sweetened, have the added benefit of being an excellent way to get fluids into your child. Mint tinctures are also available. For dosing, follow the package labeling accurately.

315

HOMEOPATHIC REMEDIES (For quick reference please refer to the "Homeopathic Remedies List" on page 32 and the inside cover.)

- A homeopathic remedy designed to decrease inflammation and fever from infections may help prevent deterioration and improve the recovery time. It can be taken 3 to 6 times daily when the virus is active (for example, fever, lethargy, etc.). (General Support 2)
- A homeopathic remedy designed to have a soothing effect on abdominal cramping may be useful. It can be given 3 to 8 times per day as needed for relief of cramping until the cramping has subsided. (Pain 1)
- A homeopathic remedy designed to reduce nausea and vomiting may be helpful. It may be given once every hour up to 10 times per day. (Digestive 4)

BACH FLOWER REMEDIES

- Rescue Remedy™ may be of use if your child is uncomfortable from the illness, stress, or anxiety. You may use 2 drops every 10 minutes to every few hours to calm restlessness as needed.
- A lukewarm bath with 10 drops of Rescue Remedy™ added to the bathwater is often very effective at relieving agitation and stress in general.

NUTRITIONALS AND SUPPLEMENTS

- Probiotics

DIETARY GUIDELINES

- The most important aspect of dietary management of vomiting is preventing dehydration, through careful fluid management. Please read and follow the guidelines in the "Home Care" section above. Once good fluid intake is established you may use the following table as a general guideline for water in addition to normal fluid intake:

AGE	OUNCES OF WATER PER DAY
2 to 5 years old	12 to 18 ounces
5 to 12 years old	18 to 24 ounces
13 and up	32 to 48 ounces

When to Call Your Health-care Provider

Call immediately if any of the following occur:
- Vomiting persists for more than 12 hours or the above measures do not work.
- Blood is present in the vomitus (not present from nosebleeds).
- Abdominal pain persists for more than 2 hours and is worsening and/or constant.
- Persistent vomiting is associated with head injury. See "Head Injury" section first.
- Signs of dehydration develop (dry mouth, marked decrease in urine output, absence of tears with crying), especially in infants. See "Dehydration" section.
- Your child under 2 years of age does not urinate for more than 8 hours and your child older than 2 years of age for more than 12 hours.
- Green bile is present in vomitus.
- Your child becomes difficult to awaken or is confused.
- There is a possibility of poisoning.
- Your child develops a fever greater than 105 degrees.

Call within 24 hours if:
- The illness is no better and signs of dehydration are beginning to develop.
- Intermittent abdominal pain continues for more than 3 days.
- Both diarrhea and vomiting are present.

 ## Other Relevant Sections

Abdominal Pain
Colic and The Fussy Baby
Dehydration
Diarrhea
Head Injury

VOMITING

Prevention

Prevention techniques are dictated by the vomiting trigger. For reflux, keep the head of the crib elevated and make sure your child is upright after feeds. It may be necessary to keep your baby in the upright position most of the day.

For infectious causes—viral, bacterial, or parasitic—meticulous hand-washing is the key. After you have handled your child's oral or nasal secretions, dirty diapers, vomitus, stools, etc., wash your hands carefully. Any contact with your ill child or objects he may have touched should be followed by hand-washing. Encourage your children to keep their hands out of their mouths.

You should also instruct your ill child and siblings to wash their hands often during an illness. Avoid exposure of your healthy child to others known to be ill with a diarrheal illness. Daycare and school will often provide information about whether a diarrheal infection is present.

Allergic triggers may be handled by identifying the exact trigger and eliminating it.

For motion sickness, avoid long car trips, especially after meals. Preferential seating in the front seat of the car may also help. You may want to medicate your child to prevent vomiting from motion sickness. See "OTC Medication Recommendations and Dosages" section.

Keep medications and household cleansers safely stored out of reach.

Description/Physiology

Warts are a very common, generally harmless childhood disease. They are viral in origin and only mildly contagious. Warts are most commonly found on the hands and feet but may occur anywhere on the body. There may be one isolated wart or dozens present. Boys are more often affected than girls. They are more of a cosmetic concern than anything else, but their location may create some discomfort and repeated irritation.

There are several wart varieties, depending on the type of virus that causes it. Warts can grow anywhere on the human body. Warts that grow on the soles of the feet are called "plantar" warts. They may be large and uncomfortable. Flat warts are small, pale, slightly raised warts that commonly grow on the face. Larger warts may occur on the hands, may grow in clusters, and may be painful. Warts that grow near the nail beds can be particularly difficult to treat. These types of warts are called "verruca vulgaris," which means "common warts." They usually have a surface that looks somewhat like cauliflower.

The other major type of wart is known as "molluscum contagiosum." These are caused by a different type of virus than the common wart. They have a more smooth and rounded surface, similar to the top of an octopus' head, which is where they get their name; "molluscum" is a scientific name for the octopus. They are usually small—1 to 3 millimeters in size—and are most commonly found on the trunk and upper extremities, though they can be found almost anywhere. This type of wart tends to spread more readily than common warts (for example, spreading from the chest to the part of the upper arm that rubs against the chest).

Wart viruses are acquired through direct skin-to-skin contact with an infected child.

Causes/Epidemiology

As mentioned, only viruses cause warts. There may be several viruses active in the community that produce warts.

There is no seasonal occurrence to warts; they can be acquired throughout the year.

Expected Course

Once a wart virus takes hold in the top skin layer (epidermis), it sends roots deeper into the skin and begins to spread out along the skin surface. Some warts remain very small while others reach a very large size. Small nearby "satellite" warts may develop, and warts may be spread anywhere else on the body, presumably by scratching.

Some wart locations are particularly uncomfortable for the child. For example, certain pressure spots on the feet may make walking uncomfortable. Warts on the hands can be frequently irritated or abraded and may often bleed. Facial warts are very visible and embarrassing.

It is rare that any secondary complications occur with warts. Once in a great while a scratched wart may become infected.

It is also very common that, if left alone, many warts will disappear. This may take a year or two. This is because the body's own immune system eventually overcomes the invading virus.

 ## Contagiousness/Immunity

The viruses that cause warts are mildly contagious. They are spread through direct skin-to-skin contact with an infected child. Some children may never develop warts despite close, repeated contact, while others are quite susceptible. Relative to other viruses, such as cold viruses, these viruses are far less contagious. In addition, having warts at any point in one's life offers no immunity later on. Children may acquire warts throughout their childhood and adolescence.

 ## Home Care

The goals for treatment at home are primarily to prevent discomfort and spreading when possible. It is safe to observe warts to determine which warts may require treatment by your health-care provider. We ask you to read through the entire "Home Care" section first to determine which of our recommendations make the most sense for your child's current situation.

1. Acid treatment. For many years the mainstay of OTC treatment of warts has been to use a solution of mild acid applied directly to the wart. There are many commercial products available, such as Occlusal®-HP. This technique is both effective and relatively painless but is also slow and

requires diligent compliance. Bathe or moisten the wart site and then pat dry. This softened tissue will more rapidly absorb the acid you are about to apply. The acid is dabbed onto the wart daily (try to keep it off the healthy surrounding skin). It should be allowed to dry, then may be covered with a light bandage. Prior to each application you may gently scrape off the top layers of the wart with a pumice stone, an emery board, or a single-edged razor blade. (Do not scrape deeply enough to draw blood.) This abrasion may help speed the removal process. Because this method can cause blistering and peeling, it should be applied by a parent or responsible teen. Since it is possible that a faint scar will develop where the wart was, we do not recommend using it on the face.

2. Acid-impregnated plaster. This is another acid method that requires daily application of an acid-impregnated adhesive plaster directly on top of the wart. One example is Mediplast®. Make sure that the plaster is only contacting the wart. The rest of the technique is identical to "Acid treatment" above.

3. Duct tape method. Cut a piece of duct tape slightly larger than the wart and apply it to the wart. Leave it in place for one week. Then remove the tape and soak the wart in water or apply a wet compress. Then gently scrape off the top layers of the wart with a pumice stone, an emery board, or a single-edged razor blade. (Do not scrape deeply enough to draw blood.) Leave the wart uncovered overnight and then reapply the tape for another week. You may repeat this process weekly, and most warts may resolve in 4 to 8 weeks.

4. Cryosurgery. If these OTC methods fail, in spite of your diligence, a visit to your health-care provider may be necessary for cryosurgery, or a "freezing" treatment. This technique involves freezing the wart with a stream of liquid nitrogen. Discomfort is variable and ranges from mild to moderate for most patients. If the pain is too intense, discontinue the treatment. The lesion may throb for several hours after the treatment and frequently the wart will form a blister that may take a few days to heal. Several treatments are usually required approximately 2 to 4 weeks apart.

5. Dermatology referral. On occasion, depending on the location, number, and type of warts, we refer patients to a dermatologist for treatment.

WARTS

 Integrated Therapies

(Please refer to the section on "Administering Integrated Treatments" on page 19 for guidance on using any of the therapies that follow.)

HERBAL REMEDIES (For quick reference please refer to the "Herbal Remedies List" on page 31 and the inside cover.)

- Echinacea/astragalus can be used to support the immune system in helping resolve a viral infection. For dosing, follow the package labeling accurately.
- Tea tree oil, for topical use only, has a natural antiviral effect. It can be used to treat warts. Apply a small drop of tea tree oil directly onto the wart (avoid getting it on the surrounding skin) and cover it with a bandage. Repeat this treatment 1 to 2 times a day until the wart is gone.

HOMEOPATHIC REMEDIES (For quick reference please refer to the "Homeopathic Remedies List" on page 32 and the inside cover.)

- Thuja is a single potency homeopathic remedy that may have beneficial effect in resolving warts. It may be given 1 to 2 times a day until the wart disappears. If no improvement is seen within 3 to 4 weeks, therapy should be discontinued.

 When to Call Your Health-care Provider

There are no emergencies involving warts. Thus, all calls regarding warts should wait until office hours.

Call within 24 hours if:
- All of the above measures have been unsuccessful over a period of several weeks.

  Be sure to tell your health-care provider exactly how many warts there are and where they are located. In some cases too many warts (more than 5) or difficult locations (such as the face, the nail beds, or the genitals) will require a dermatologist's evaluation and treatment.
- A wart is scratched and appears infected with a large red area spreading around the wart.

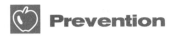 Prevention

Encourage your children to wash their hands often, especially after playing with other children with warts. Avoid direct contact with a wart whenever possible. When your child has a wart, encourage him not to pick or scratch it.

Jerry Rubin, M.D.

Dr. Rubin's areas of special interest are behavior management and holistic medicine. Dr. Rubin graduated from the University of Utah medical school in 1977, completing his pediatric internship and residency at the University of Colorado Health Sciences Center, after which he joined Dr. Klein in practice.

Dean Prina, M.D.

Dr. Prina's areas of special interest are the newborn, special-needs children, writing educational materials and holistic care. Dr. Prina graduated from medical school at the University of California, San Diego in 1979, completing his pediatric internship and residency at the University of Colorado Health Sciences Center. He joined Partners in Pediatrics in 1982.

Nancy Broady Lataitis, M.D.

Dr. Lataitis' areas of special interest are the adolescent, asthma, and special-needs newborns. Dr. Lataitis graduated from Vanderbilt University medical school in 1984, completing her pediatric internship and residency at the University of Colorado Health Sciences Center. She joined Partners in Pediatrics in 1987.

Jordan R. Klein, M.D.

Dr. Klein's areas of special interest are allergy and asthma. Dr. Klein graduated from the University of Louisville medical school in 1974, completing his pediatric internship and residency at the University of Miami in 1977. In that same year, he moved to Denver and established his pediatric practice.

To share "Naturally Healthy Kids"

with friends, family and associates,

or to order additional copies for yourself,

go to our website

www.naturallyhealthykids.com

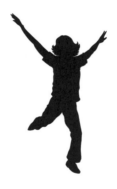